Nail Art
SOURCEBOOK

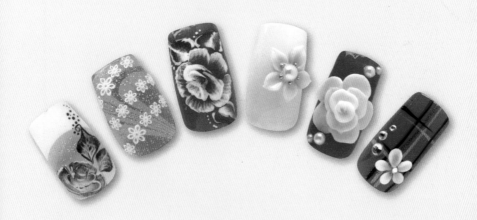

THIS IS A CARLTON BOOK

Published in 2012 by Carlton Books Limited
20 Mortimer Street
London W1T 3JW

10 9 8 7 6 5 4 3 2 1

Text, Design and Special Photography © 2012
Carlton Books Limited 2012

Some of the material in this book was previously
published in *Nail Art* by Pansy Alexander, ©
Carlton Books 1999.

A CIP catalogue record for this book is available
from the British Library.

ISBN 978 1 78097 089 9
Senior Executive Editor: Lisa Dyer
Managing Art Director: Lucy Coley
Copy Editor: Lara Maiklem
Designer: Anna Pow
Picture Research: Jenny Meredith
Production: Maria Petalidou
Photography by Karl Andersen
Front Cover by Lucy Coley

Printed in China

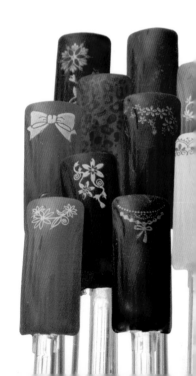

Nail Art
SOURCEBOOK

Pansy Alexander-Potter
& Mineko Sugita

CARLTON

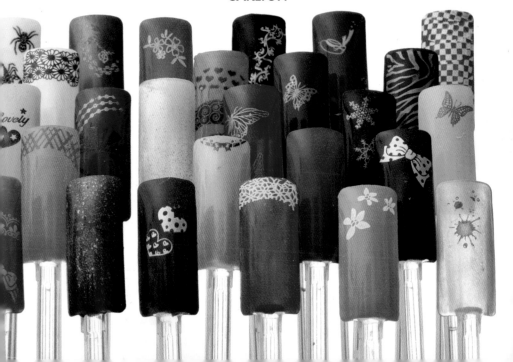

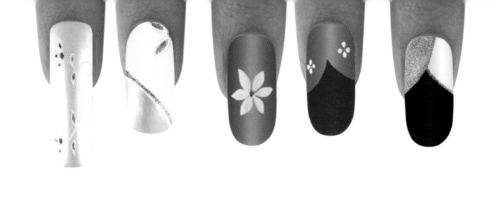
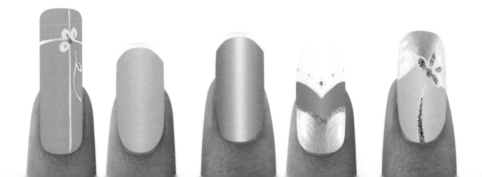

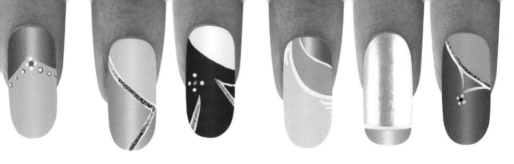

Contents

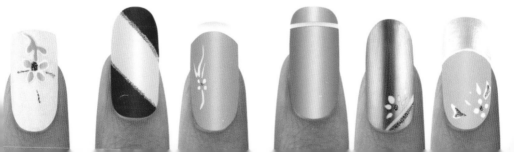

Introduction

Nail art is a fabulous way to create new looks for your fingertips and allows you to have fun experimenting with patterns and colours, treating your nails as a blank canvas. The following collection of over 500 designs is based on current fashion trends and lets you choose designs to take to the salon or do at home. All the techniques you need to create amazing talons are illustrated in the following pages. The introduction explains the basic techniques to creating your own designs, including a list of the materials you'll need – the different coloured nail polishes, gels and paints and advice on the types of brushes you should use, together with any transfers, striping tape, stick-on designs or gemstones.

Your basic nail-art kit should include a good range of nail polishes and water-based paints in various colours, a selection of brushes and a special-effects tool, together with striping tape, transfers, stencils, gemstone secures and nail-art sealer to protect your finished designs. For filling in large areas of colour, use nail polish, and for adding more intricate details, use water-based paints applied with a very fine paint brush; if you want to paint perfect straight lines, use a striping brush (see page 12).

Whether you choose to copy the designs on the following pages, use them as inspiration for your own versions, or take them to a nail technician to have the design professionally executed, there are hundreds of ideas here to help you to get a look you will love.

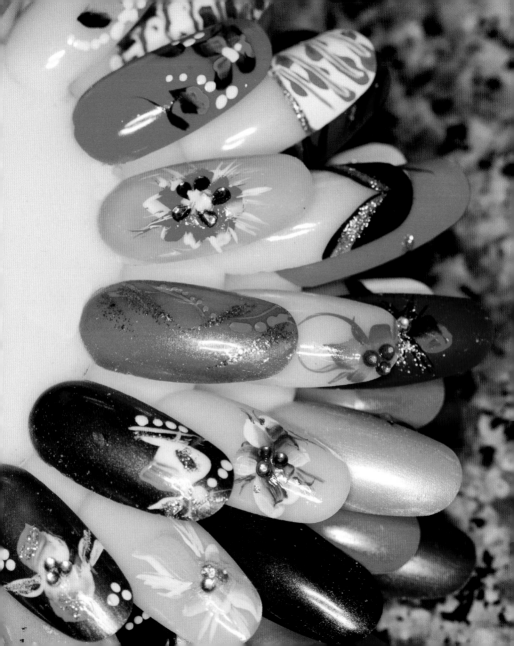

Artificial Nails and Tips

Plastic press-on nail are ideal if your own nails aren't long enough to paint. They cover the natural nail and are shaped to fit under the cuticle. They are either flat or curved, with square, round or oval tips. You can paint the design before applying them, buy them in different colours and finishes, and you can also use them to practise your nail art.

You can also use nail tips to extend your natural nails; these are glued onto the top third of the nail and then filed to blend with your natural nail bed. Nail tips need to be custom-fit to your nail as they will not be an exact fit. To do this, select a slightly larger rather than a slightly smaller tip and file the side edges to create a perfect fit. To apply:

- Select the correct size, making sure they fit over the entire nail, or file to fit.
- Place a drop of glue on the underside of the tip in the "well", press firmly to the nail and hold for 30 seconds. If the glue comes in contact with the skin, use an acetone-based remover to melt it away.
- Using tip cutters, cut the tips to the desired length and shape the free edge.
- File the join and buff until smooth.
- Never pull the tips off; use an acetone-based polish remover to soak and loosen the nail tip.

Caring for your Nails

Keeping your hands and cuticles moisturized and nourished is the key to having soft hands and healthy, strong nails. Here are a few simple procedures you can follow to keep them in peak condition:

- Always dry your hands thoroughly when you wash them.
- Use a moisturizing hand lotion regularly and massage it well into the skin, especially around the cuticles.
- Wear protective gloves when using cleaning products.
- Use a non-acetone nail-polish remover, but don't use it more than once a week as this will strip and weaken the nails.
- Remember not to file your nails more than necessary, and always work in one direction to avoid weakening the nails.

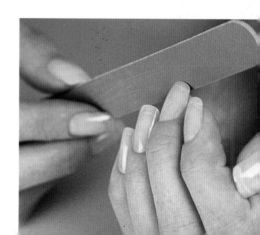

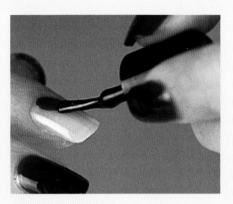

Conditioning Manicure

You don't have to visit a salon to have gorgeous pampered nails. It takes just a few minutes to perform a basic mini-manicure at home. Try to do the following once a month to keep your nails in top condition:

- Massage the skin around the nail using a good cuticle cream, then soak the fingers in warm water with a soap-free cleanser for 1–2 minutes.
- Wrap the end of an orange-wood stick with cotton wool. Dip it in the warm water and gently rub the edges of the nail plate to remove any dead cuticle.
- Dry the hands thoroughly and apply some nourishing hand cream, massaging it in well.

- Working in one direction, shape your nails into rounded, square or "squoval" tips, using a soft to normal emery board – if the emery board is too hard, it will cause flaking and chipping at the edge of the nail. Never use an emery board across the surface of the nail plate.
- To prevent coloured polish from staining your nails, and to help strengthen them and smooth ridges, always apply two coats of an all-in-one conditioning base coat, strengthener and top coat first.
- Paint your nails with two coats of polish, allowing each coat to dry naturally before applying the next.
- Apply a top coat of clear varnish to seal the colour and help prevent chipping. Refresh your nails every other day with a further coat of top glaze.

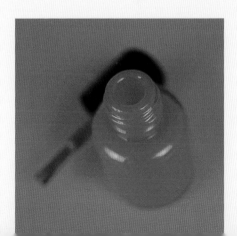

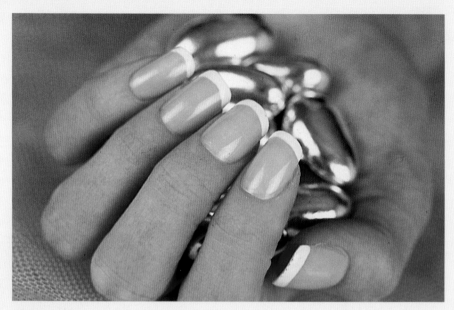

Basic French Manicure

A French manicure uses a flesh-pink base and white polish for the tip. For a similar effect, an American manicure substitutes a beige base for the pink.

- Over a base coat, apply two coats of natural-looking flesh-pink polish and, while it is still tacky, lay a length of damp cotton on the tips of the nails to mark a guideline for the edge of the white area; remove the cotton and let the polish dry.
- Define the tips with two coats of white polish and let it dry.
- Finish by applying a top coat of nail-art sealer to the nail.

Nail Polishes

Nail polish comes in a vast array of fabulous colours from classic flat colours, to up-to-the-minute metallic, pearlized and iridescent shades, including two-tone polishes and glitter varnishes that are great for parties. You will need a good range of your favourite nail polishes to act as base colours for your designs. In addition to the prerequisite reds and pinks, you should have nail polishes in black, white, green, blue and yellow. For special effects, you should have gold and silver metallic polishes and a couple of glitter polishes.

Always buy small bottles of nail polish, since larger bottles become sticky and unusable after they have been around for a while. You should also always make sure you clean the rims of the bottles after using them to make sure you don't transfer dried flakes of polish onto the nails when you paint them.

First, shake the bottle or roll it between your palms to mix the polish. Take care not to overload the brush. Apply the first coat by making one stroke down the centre of the nail, then apply a single stroke to each side. Avoid touching the cuticle area with polish by leaving a thin line around the edge of the nail. Let it dry naturally and when it is completely dry apply a second coat to achieve smooth coverage without streaking.

Acrylic Gels

For 3D nail art you can purchase gel powder in pots or paints in tubes or pens; the latter are good for drawing lines and creating dots. A fine brush can be used for more detailed designs.

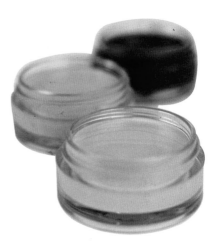

Nail Paints

These acrylic, water-based, non-toxic, quick-drying paints can be used to add pattern and detail to a nail polish base. A huge range of colours are available, including opalescents and fluorescents – opalescents are pearl-white, but when used sparingly on a dark nail polish they become very vibrant. To begin with you should at least have white, red, blue, green and yellow paints, since they can be mixed to create other colours and shades. Place a small drop of paint on a palette and close the jar to keep it fresh. Always try to keep the lid and rim clean and apply paint sparingly, using a fine brush.

Nail-Art Brushes

Brushes should be used to apply nail paints, and you should have at least three of the following in your nail-art kit:

- Standard brush for creating the main features of your design.
- Fine-detail brush, with short bristles that taper to a very fine tip, for intricate work.
- Striping brush with long, even bristles for creating straight, well-defined lines or stripes.
- Fan brush with flat, fan-shaped bristles for feathering and other special effects.
- Special-effects tool, with a small, rounded metal tip for dotting, marbling and other special effects.

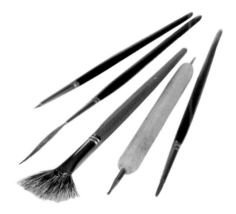

Nail Transfers

Transfers come either as individual pictures or a series of images that can be combined to create a larger design that runs across all the nails on one hand. To apply transfers:

- Apply two coats of base polish and allow your nails to completely dry.
- Cut out the image, leaving just enough room around the edge of the transfer to hold it by.
- Apply a little water to the back of the transfer and wait for 30 seconds before sliding the design off the backing and onto the nail. Press the transfer gently to make sure it is dry and lying flat.
- Add a top coat of protective nail-art sealer to finish.

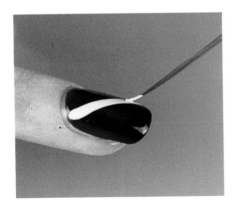

Stick-Ons

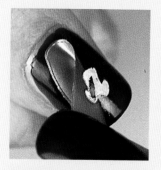

Stick-on decals, foils, motifs and bindis are easy and quick to apply. Also available are patterns in self-adhesive sheets (or wraps), which can be cut to size and simply stuck onto the nail.

- Lay the self-adhesive sheet in position over the nail and, using an orange-wood stick, mark the outline of the nail, following the curve of the cuticle.
- Carefully cut out the shape, remove the backing, and stick the pattern onto the nail, making sure it is lying flat with no air bubbles.
- Add a top coat of protective nail-art sealer.

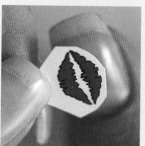

Stencils (left, top), transfers (left and below right) and stick-on sheets (below left) can be used to add ready-made decoration to nails.

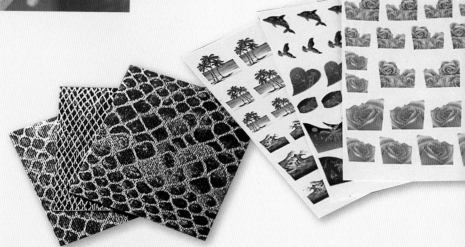

Stencils

Reusable stencils are a simple way of creating nice clean patterns. They are available in a range of designs, or you can create your own stencils by cutting tiny shapes out of a sheet of flexible card using a craft knife.

1 Apply two coats of your chosen base polish colour and allow it to completely dry.

2 Position the stencil and make sure it sits flat across the nail to keep the edges of the design clean.

3 Hold the stencil still and apply a small amount of polish through the cut-out shapes. Allow the polish to dry slightly before removing it.

4 Finish with a clear top coat.

Striping Tape

Self-adhesive striping tape can be used to enhance designs or as a guide for painting straight lines. It comes in various colours and widths, from less than 1 mm wide to a wider tape that incorporates patterns, such as squares, hearts or diamonds.

1 Apply two coats of your chosen base polish and allow your nails to dry completely.

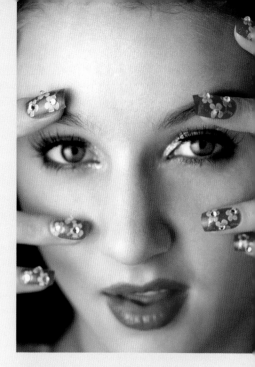

Enhance your designs with glue-on diamantés. Be sure to apply false nails to the natural nail first before coating with a gel sealer, as the nail forms will harden once sealer is applied.

2 Lay the tape over the nail in your desired pattern. Allow the ends to overhang the edge of the nail.

3 Press the tape down and trim the ends.

4 Cover the entire nail area with a top coat or clear sealer to protect the design.

Gemstones

For glamour and sparkle, incorporate rhinestones or polish secures – tiny stones, gems, studs and jewels – into your designs. These are available in a wide range of shapes, style and colours, including foil motifs such as stars, hearts and circles. To apply gemstones:

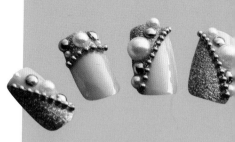

1 Apply two coats of polish. When it is dry, apply a coat of clear varnish where you want to put the decoration.

2 Position the gemstones on the wet polish. As the polish dries, they will set in place.

3 To position stones in a straight line, lay a piece of damp cotton across the wet polish to create a guideline. Remove the cotton and place the stones on the wet polish, following the line.

4 Cover the nail with a top coat of protective sealer.

Nail-Art Sealer

Water-based nail paints, striping tape, stick-on designs and transfers will readily come off when you wash your hands unless they are protected by a top coat. Any nail polish protector or top-coat glaze will seal these elements. Specialized sealer is heavier than a standard top coat, however, and should always be used when gemstones are incorporated into a design to help prevent them from coming loose from the nail.

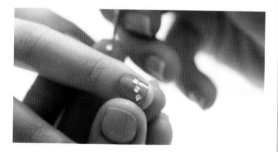

A tweezer will help you position and build up your decoration. For built-up designs, like those top left, it is easiest to work on false nails rather than the natural nail.

Complicated Designs

If you are layering paints and special effects, such as glitter, stones, and even 3D work, you need to separate out each technique and work from the large basic shapes to increasingly more detailed work. An example is shown here:

1 First paint in your basic underlying shape. Here, the heart is outlined and the surrounding area painted white, with the heart remaining the natural nail colour. Paint several layers of white to build a strong opaque colour.

2 Add thin black lines, following the curve of the bottom of the heart, then enhance it by adding white paint as a shadow. This will lift the black and bring it into relief.

3 Continue painting the details of the design, allowing the colour to dry each time so that it doesn't smudge.

4 Finish by gluing on diamanté jewels using nail adhesive, and finish with several coats of sealer.

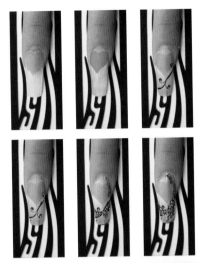

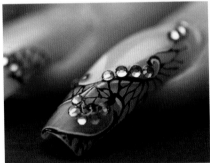

The final design has a trompe-l'oeil effect, as the bright white lines make the black stand out. You might prefer to use a black nail-art pen to do the detail work, rather than a fine-tipped brush.

Three-Dimensional Work

For this type of nail art you will need ready-made, acrylic 3D gels in a variety of colours. Alternatively, you can mix your own colours by combining clear 3D acrylic gel with different powder colours to get your own bespoke shades. For long-lasting results you can use a UV lamp to "cure" the gel, but it is also fine to just finish with several coats of sealer.

- Prepare the base with a layer of base gel, keeping a thin margin around the nail so the gel doesn't touch the skin and cuticle.
- Arrange iridescent flakes, loose glitter or any other decoration you choose by placing them in position on the wet base gel. Build up the nail with more acrylic gel along the centre.
- The shape of your nails can be refined and scratches smoothed out using a very fine nail file or white block, but remember to remove any dust before you add further layers.

- To create flowers and other designs, apply a small bead of 3D gel to the nail, press it down slightly and manipulate it with the point of the brush to create shapes. Flower petals are created by arranging circles together, and other shapes can be created by pressing the circles into hearts, diamonds or any other shapes you like.
- Build up your layers by finishing with more glitter or by attaching diamantés with nail adhesive.

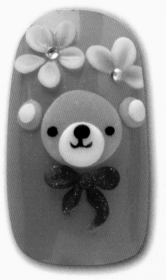
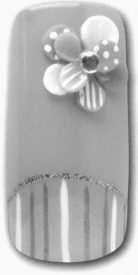

Floral Designs

Flowers, leaves and tendrils are some of the easiest designs to try first if you are a novice; flowers can be created by using dots of paint to create the petals, with a dot or diamanté glued in the centre. Try simple designs first, and build up in complexity by adding more details as well as shading or blending.

You can create dots of varying sizes by using thinner- or thicker-tipped tools, such as a striper brush, cocktail stick or pin. Lightly dip the implement into the desired colour and then dot it onto the nail, manipulate the dots as desired. Use a dragging action with your tool to create a teardrop shape for petals, or "rays" from a large dot. Alternatively, paint an outline of the flower first, then fill it in with blocks of colour, adding shading and details at later stages.

Stems can be created by painting a thin, curved green line leading to the flower, with simple leaves or thorns pointing away from the stem. You can also make thin "flicks" with a striping brush to create leaves and tendrils. To make floral designs more exciting and dramatic, try to use unusual colours, such as neons or purples and blacks, rather than just the shades you see in nature.

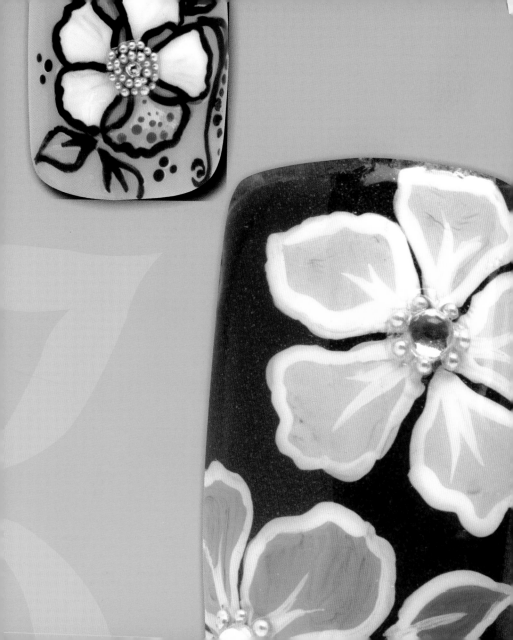

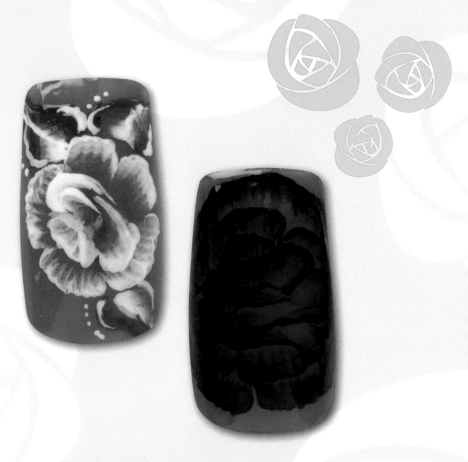

If you lack the skill to paint flowers freehand, as in these nail designs, you can "cheat" by combining stencils or transfers with hand-painted details.

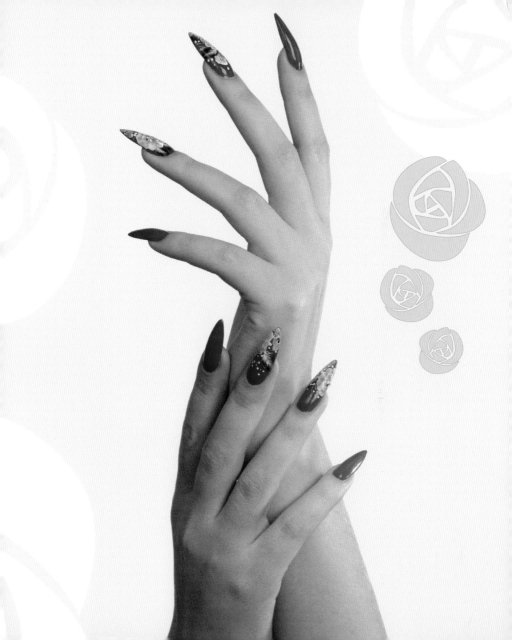

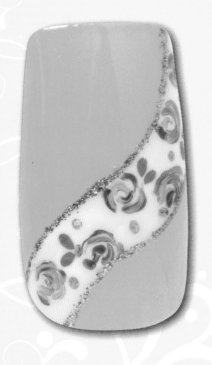

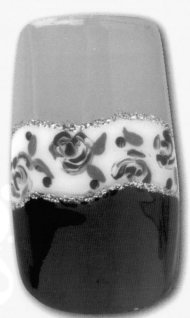

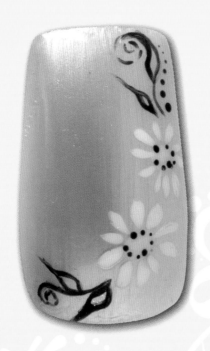
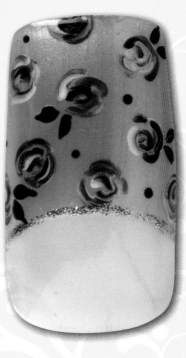

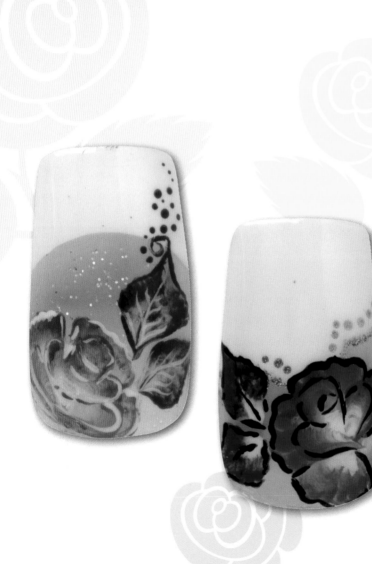

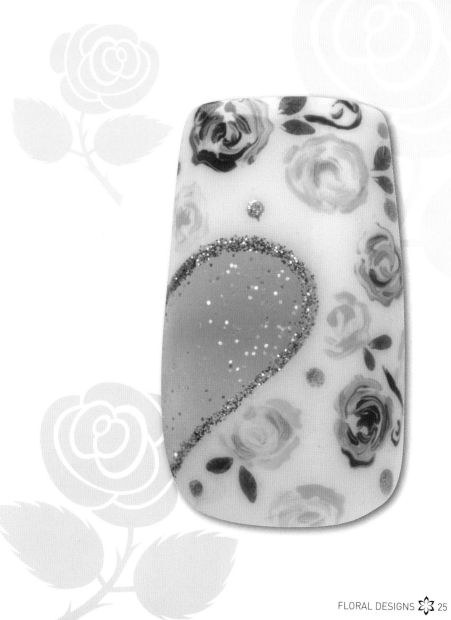

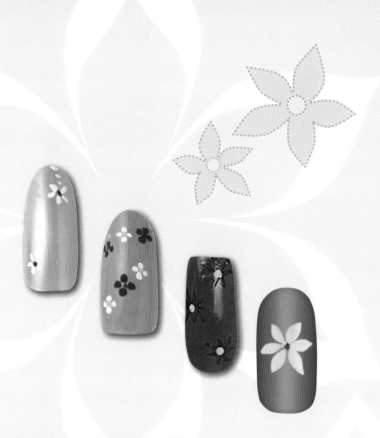

Easy flower shapes can be created by painting asterisk or star shapes and adding a central spot in a different colour, or by joining up small dots to form petals.

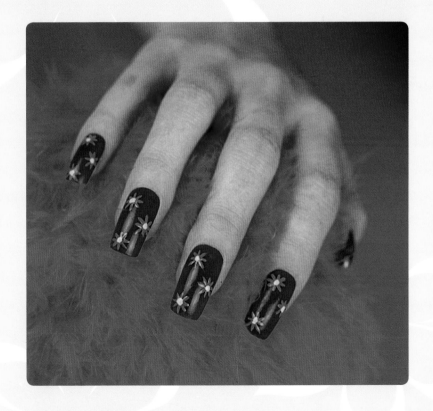

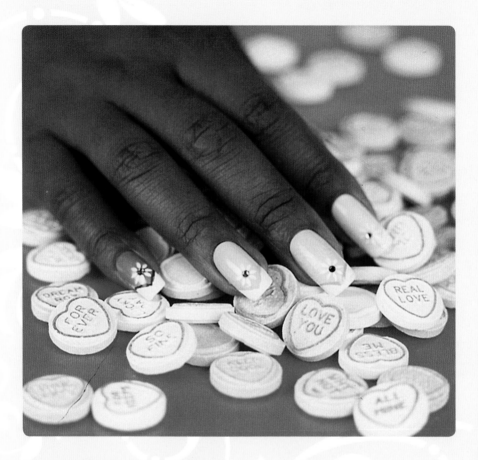

Glue a diamanté to the centre of your flowers
for extra sparkle, or add a touch of glitter for
a more subtle effect.

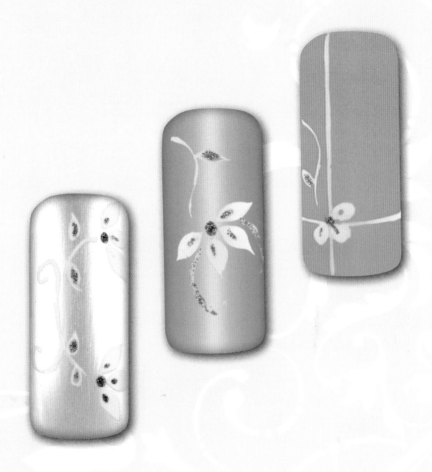

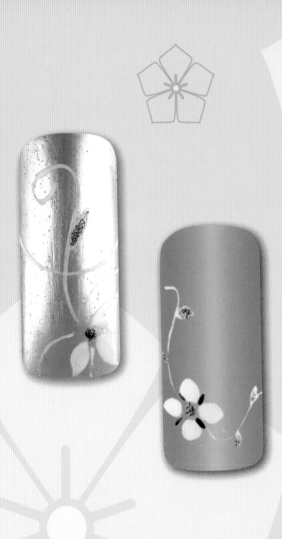
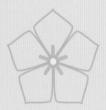

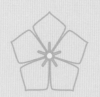

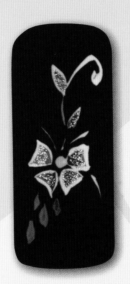

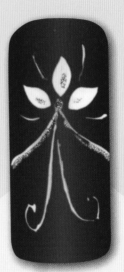

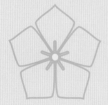

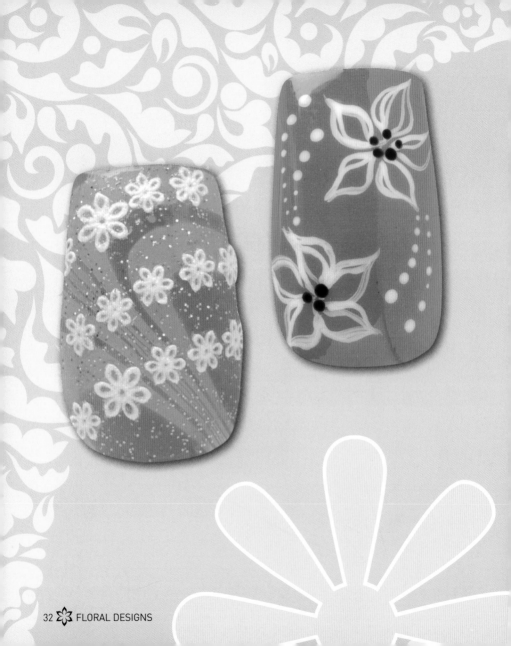

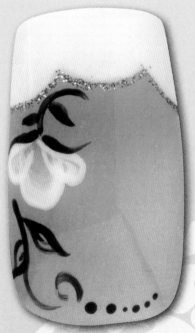
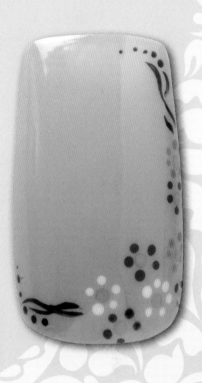

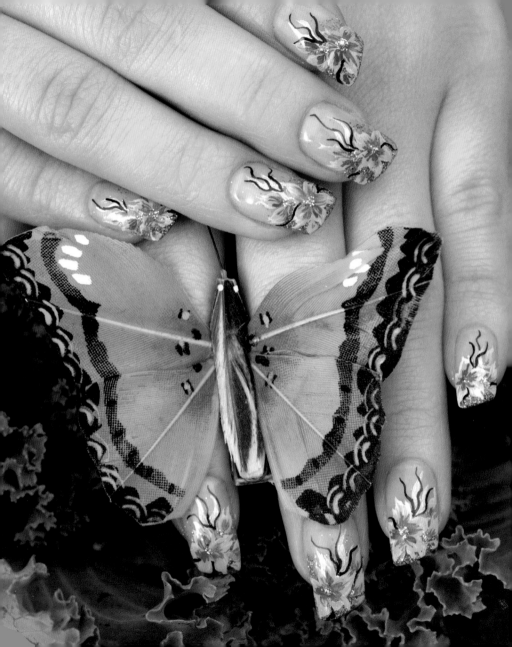

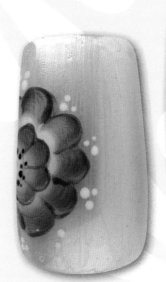

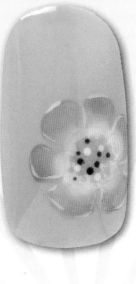

Arrange your design so that the flower is off-centre or only a part of the flower is showing. This creates a far more effective and prettier composition.

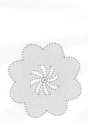

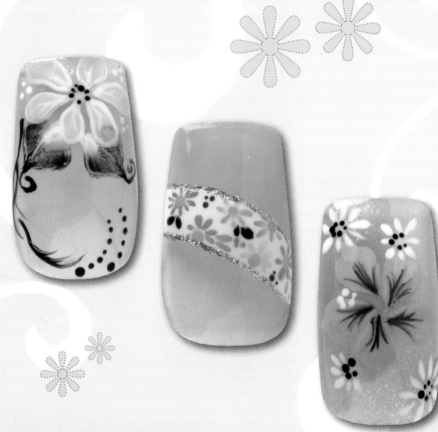

If you don't have a special-effects tool, you can use a pin, cocktail stick or even a Biro dipped in paint to add details and swirls.

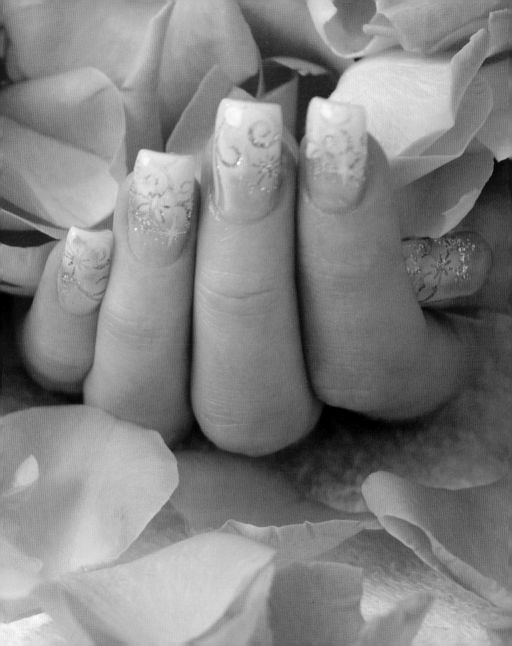

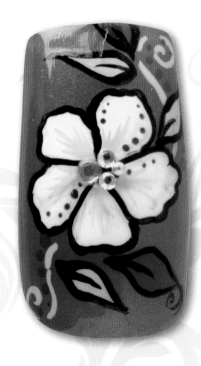

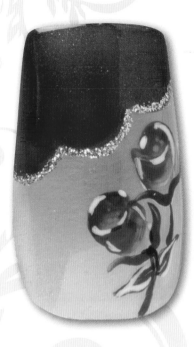

A two-colour base can make a strong background for some designs. The join doesn't need to be perfect, as you can use glitter to delineate between the two areas (above), or place your floral design on top of the join (opposite left).

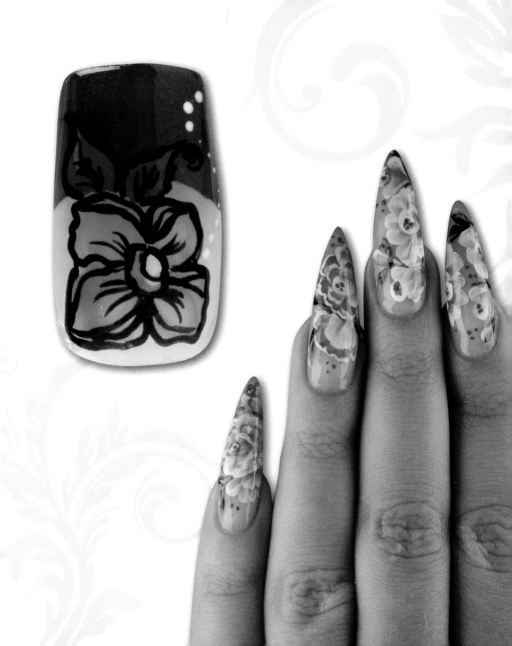

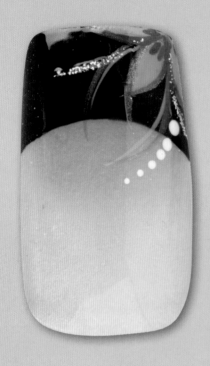

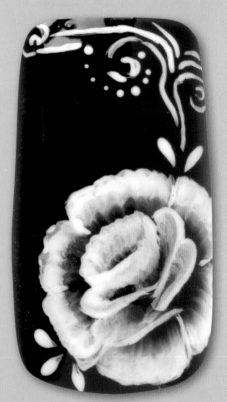

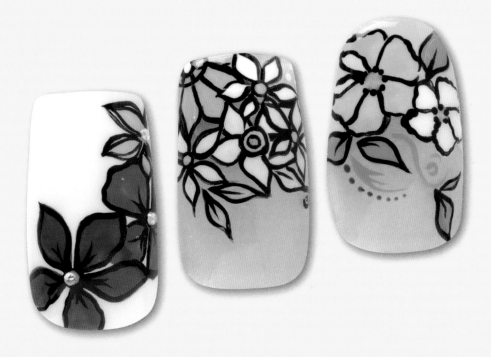

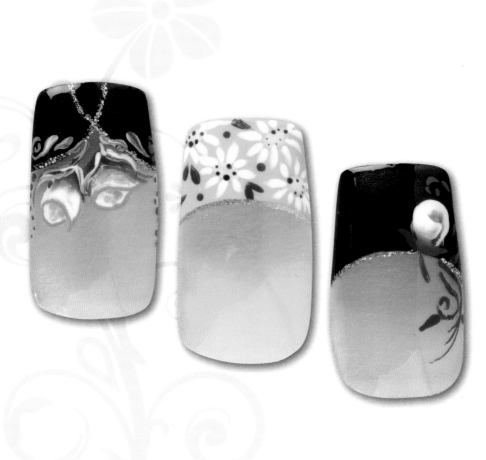

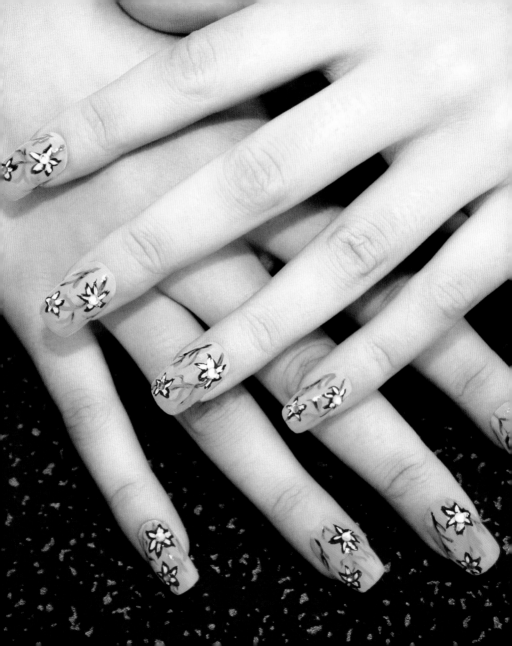

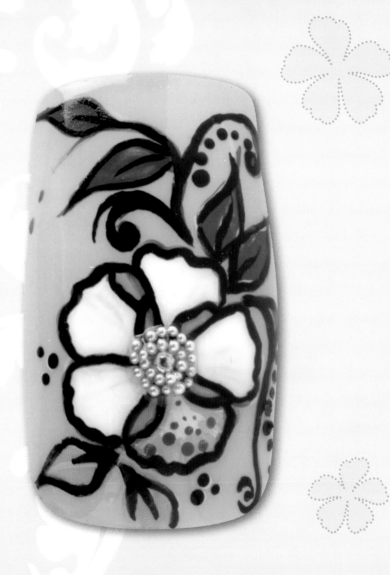

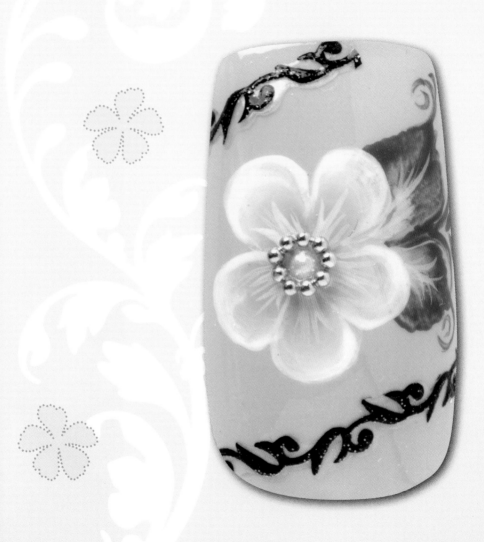

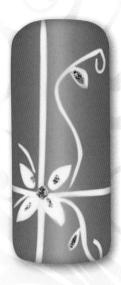
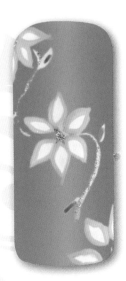
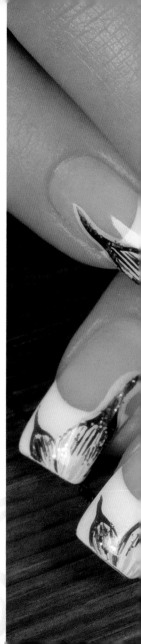

The orchid design (opposite) was first painted
in lighter pink for the petals, with purple
details added later with a fine paintbrush.
It was finished with a white outline.

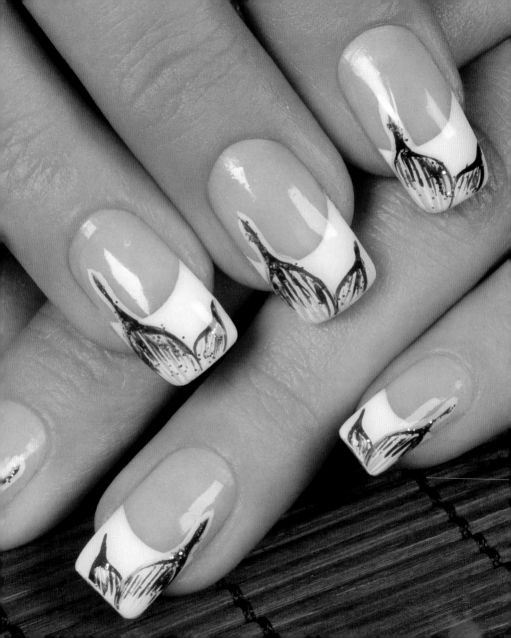

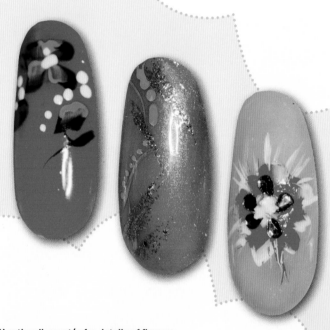

Use tiny diamantés for details of flowers,
such as the stamens on the lilies, opposite.
Groupings of odd numbers, such as three, will
always look better than using even numbers,
unless you are creating a geometric design.

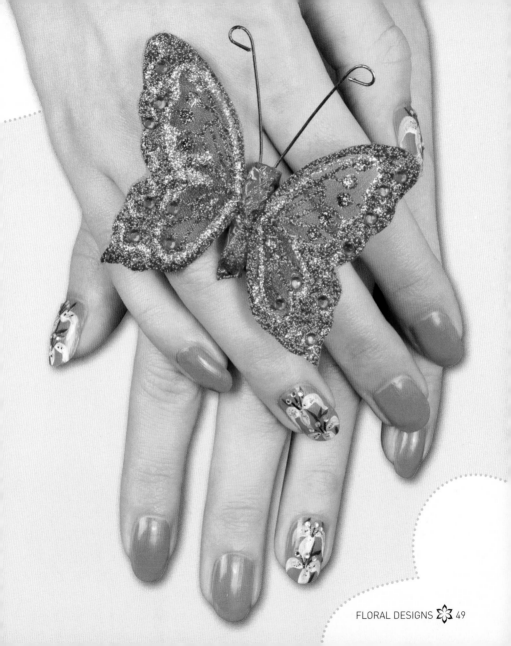

It is very easy to smudge your art, especially with intricate designs that involve many coats of colour. Always make sure each colour is fully dry before applying another, unless you are blending colours.

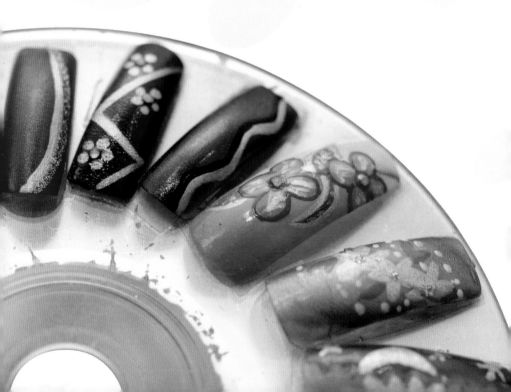

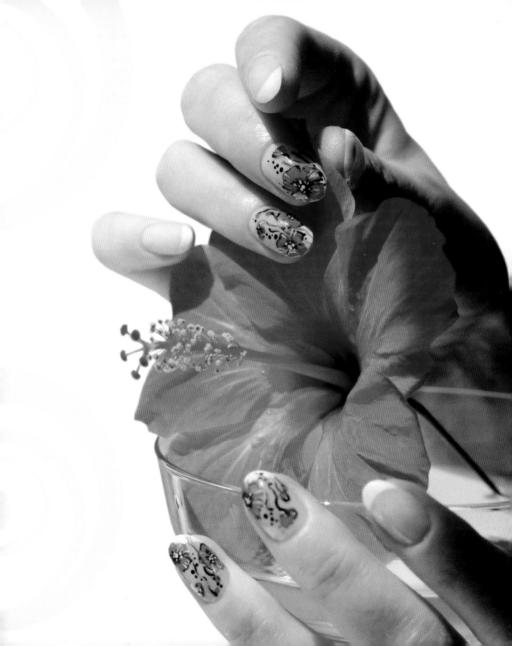

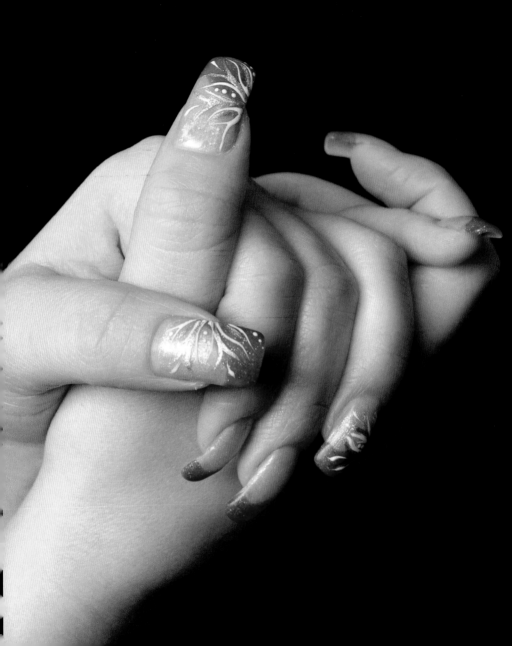

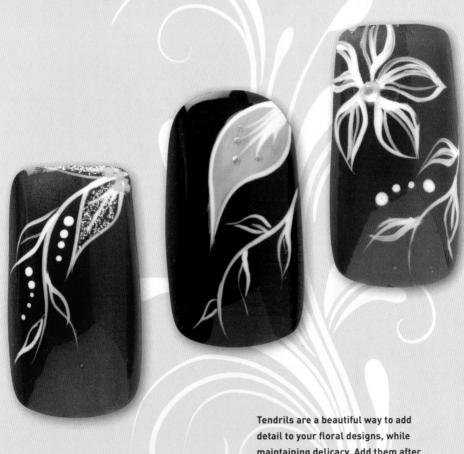

Tendrils are a beautiful way to add detail to your floral designs, while maintaining delicacy. Add them after you have completed the main flower, and position them to echo the shape and curves of the petals.

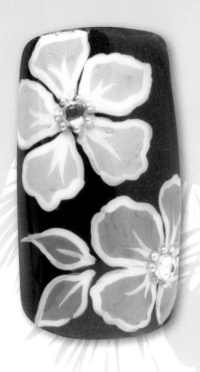
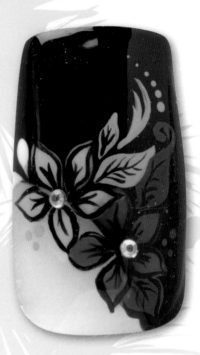

Bold colours can be set off and made more
striking by heavy outlining in black or white.
Always paint the base ("ground") colour
first, before tracing around the shapes.

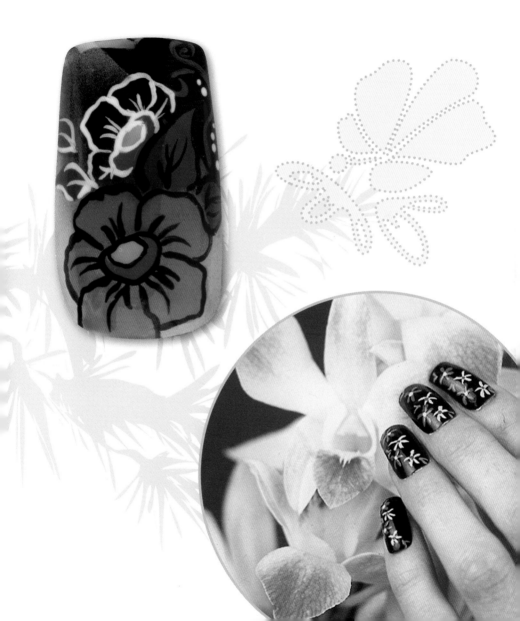

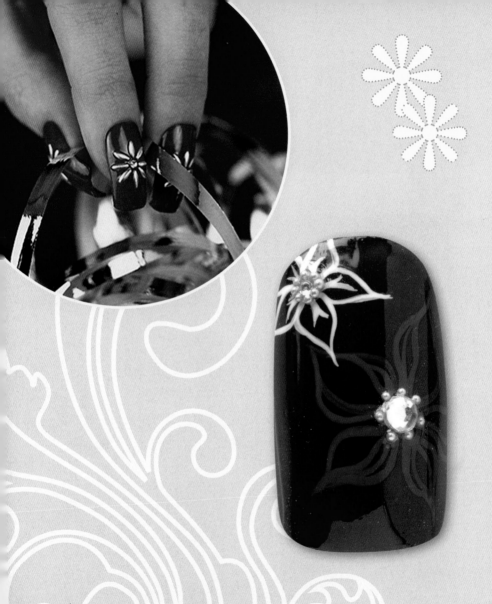

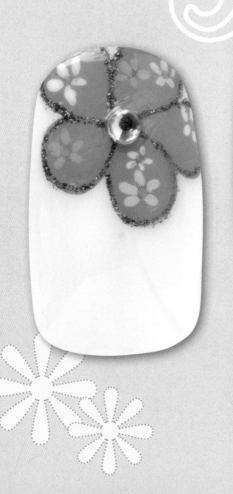

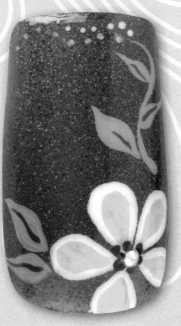

There are countless ways to create flower petals. You can make them from metal ovals and rhinestones (opposite top), or from painting teardrop shapes that radiate inward or outward.

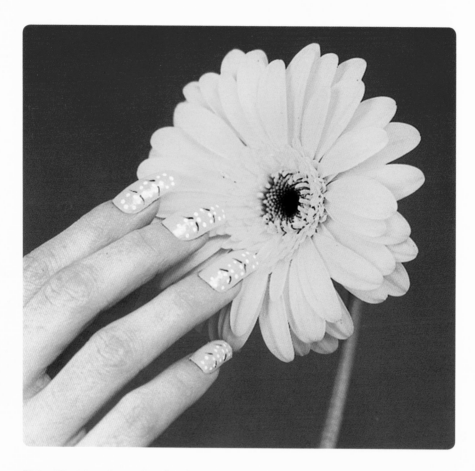

Plain white dots and green lines have been
used to represent flowers (above), while rose
transfers, layered on top of a red base coat,
creates a more elaborate floral design (right).

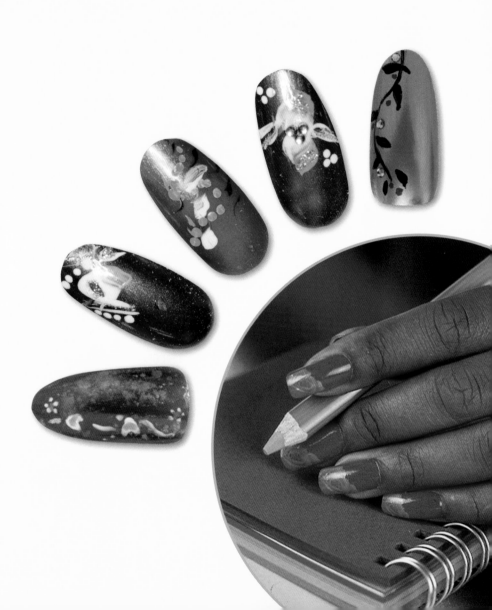

Graphic Designs

Once you've mastered straight lines, squares, squiggles and circles, you can create any number of abstract and graphic designs of varying complexity. If you find it very difficult to achieve straight-edged geometric shapes, use a peel-off stencil, sticker or striping tape to help. Nail wraps are a simple way to achieve all-over patterns quickly – they are available in checkerboard, diamond, tartan, striped and many more varieties.

For inspiration, look at Op Art to create designs like targets (bull's-eyes), chevrons, checks and stripes. The work of Bridget Riley, Victor Vasarely and Gerhard Richter can give you lots of ideas about how to use colours and geometric shapes. Experiment with repeating patterns, but give them an edge by using several different sizes. One easy way to do this with circles is to make trailing dots: simply dip a cocktail stick in the paint once and apply several dots in a row, without reapplying the colour. The dots will become smaller as less paint remains on the stick. Also try a paint-splatter look, à la Jackson Pollock, or graffiti and spray-paint effects.

Look at textile prints too – many have patterns, stars, skulls or other icons that translate well into nail art – as well as logos from fashion houses, such as the Louis Vuitton monogram or Burberry tartan.

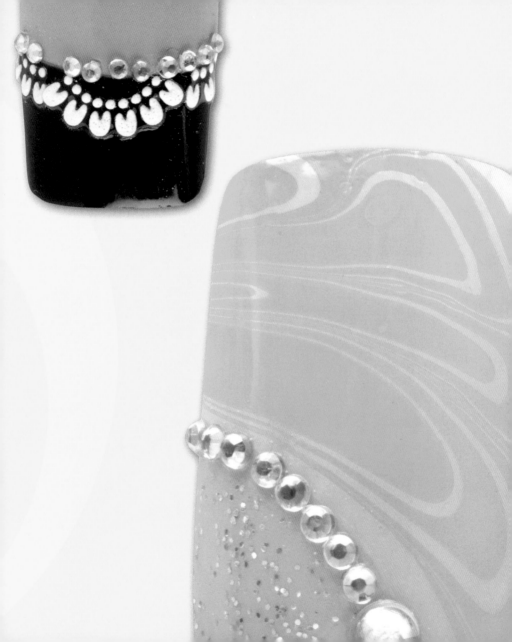

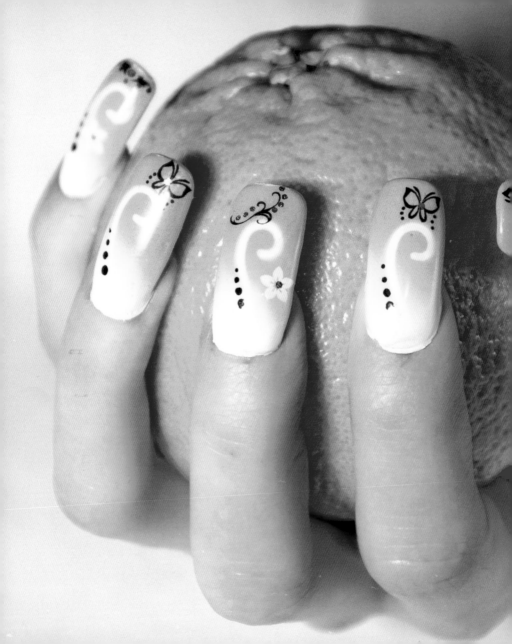

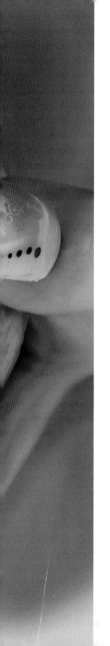

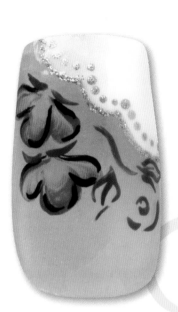

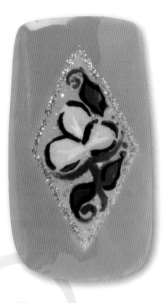

Don't worry if your designs don't match
on all fingertips – it's actually far more
interesting when they vary slightly so long
as they keep to the same colour scheme or
have similar design elements.

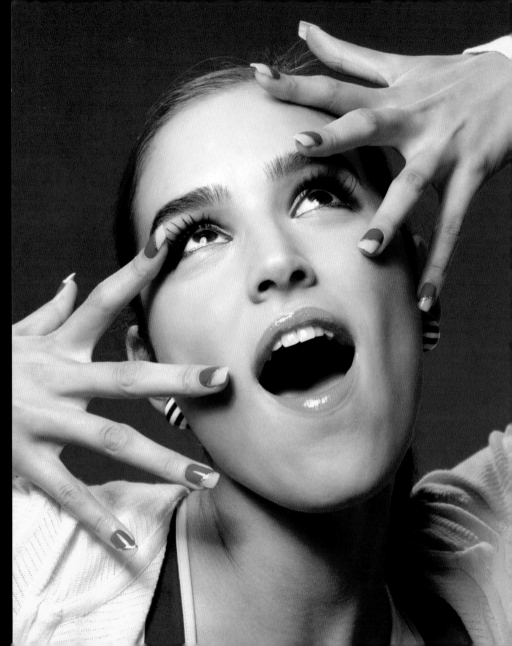

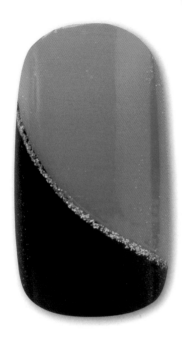

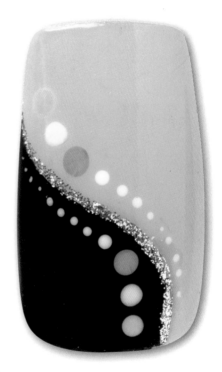

Using just two bold colours for a design can make a powerful statement. In all these artworks, the colour field has been divided in two, with further decoration added along the join.

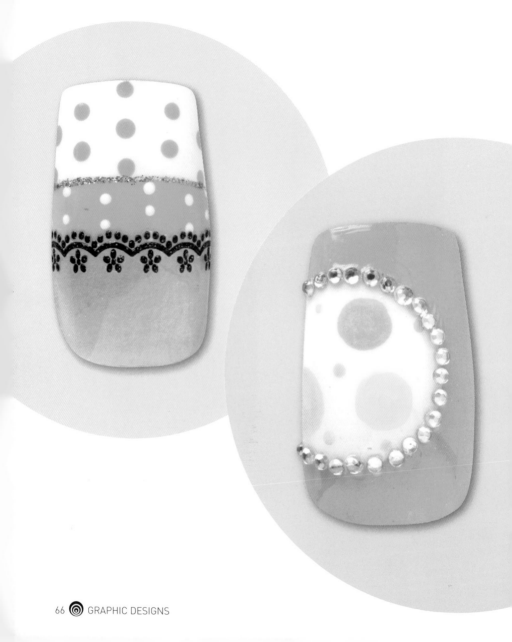

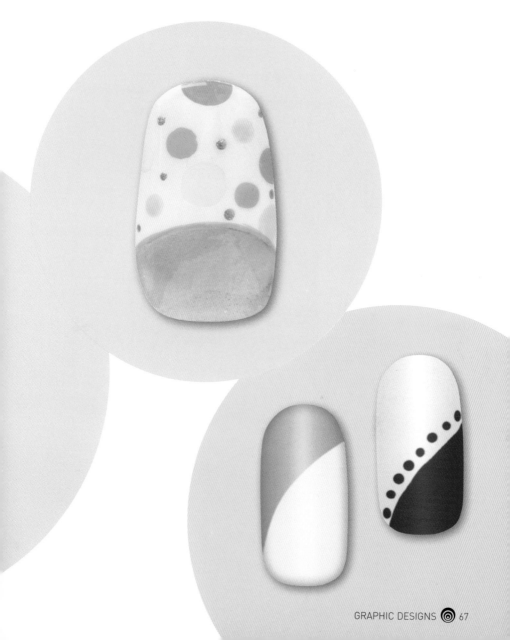

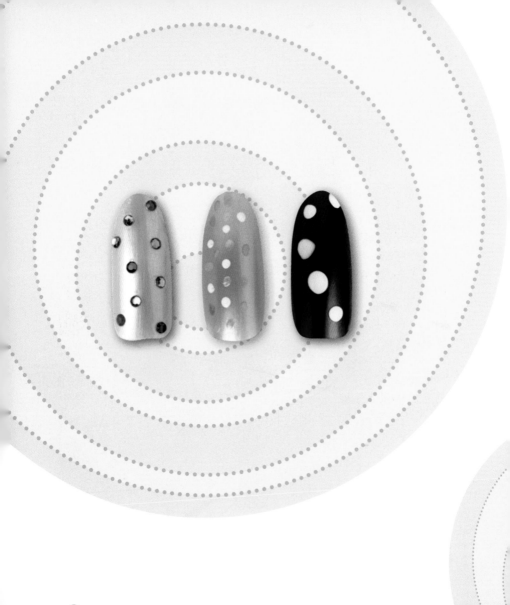

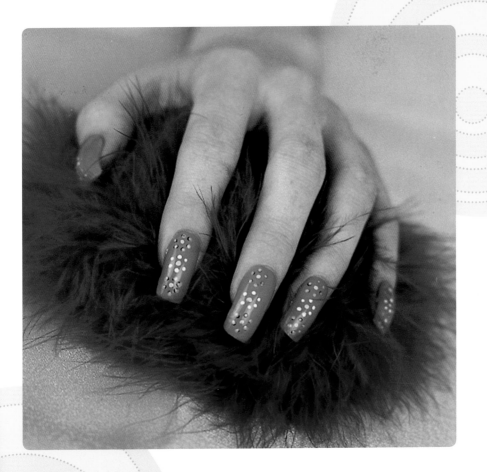

Experiment with spotty designs by varying
the size of the dots or by placing dots
randomly or in rows. To create a sparkling
effect, use round coloured gemstones
instead of paint for the dots.

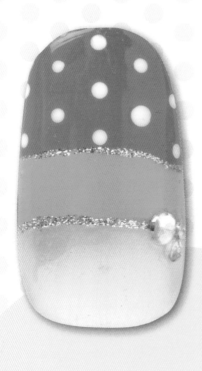
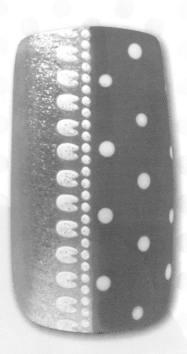

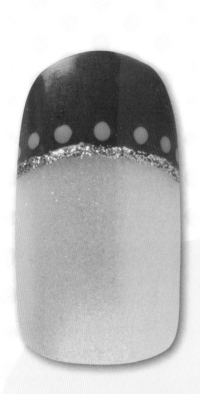
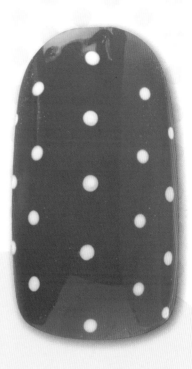

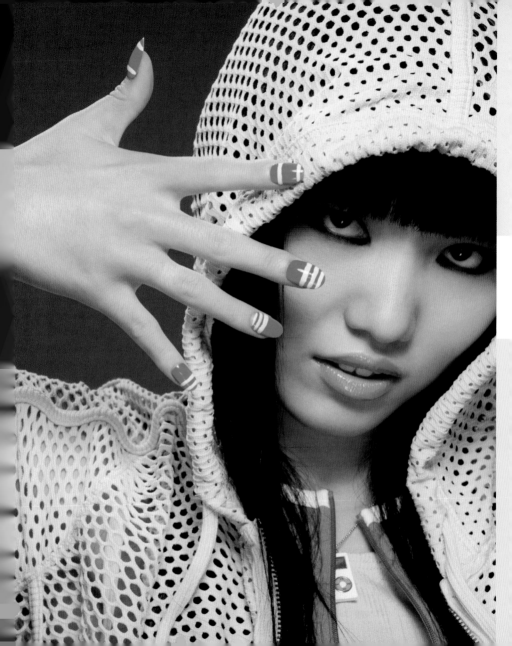

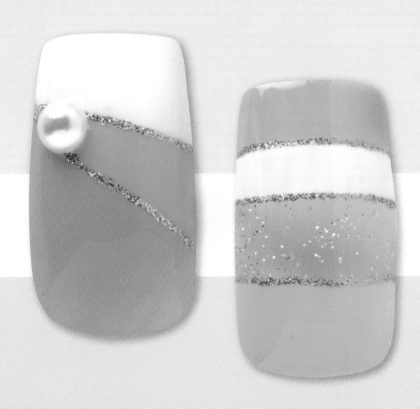

Wavy and uneven stripes make a more
interesting design than keeping each
nail exactly the same. Mix it up with both
horizontal and vertical lines.

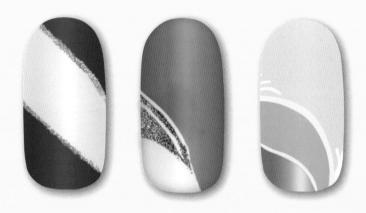

A striping brush is useful to paint narrow horizontal stripes across the nail, but you could also use an eyeliner or fine-tipped brush. When alternating colours, make sure you use separate tools, or wash the tool between colours.

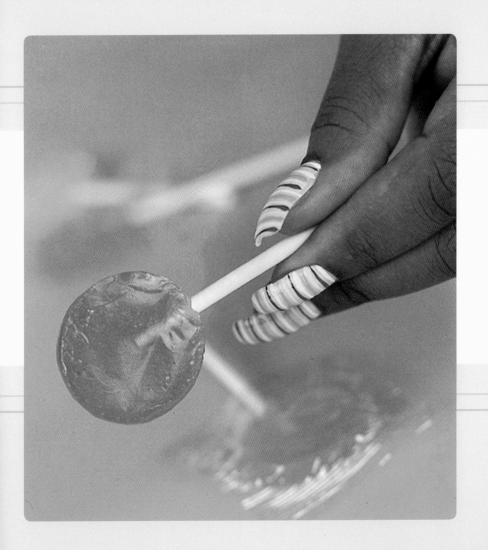

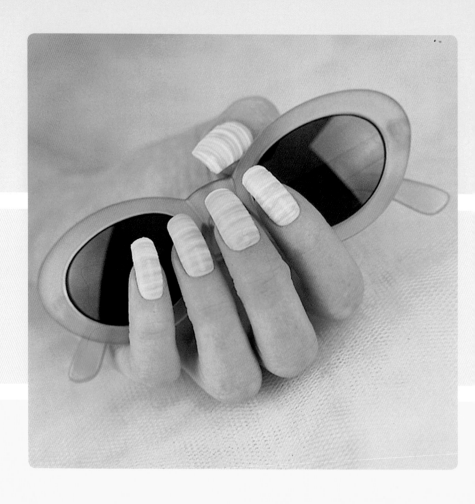

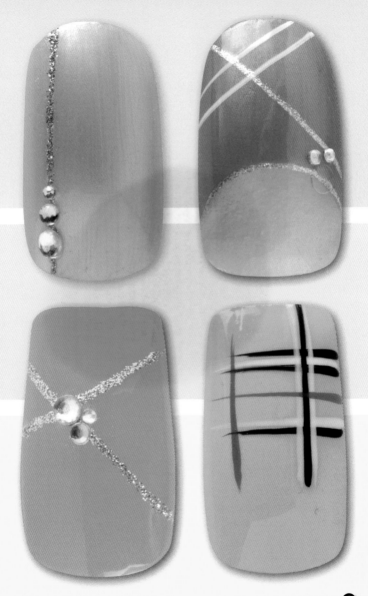

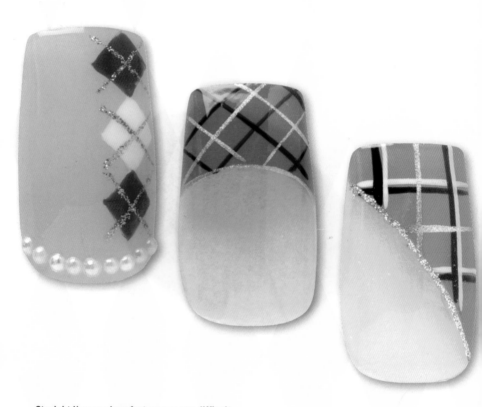

Straight lines and perfect curves are difficult
to achieve freehand. To make it easier, use
peel-off striping tape or low-tack household
masking tape to create a clean line.

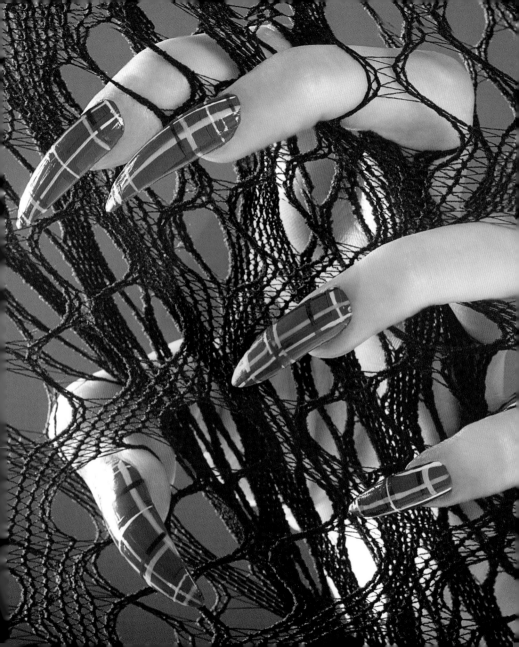

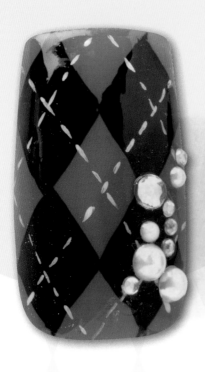
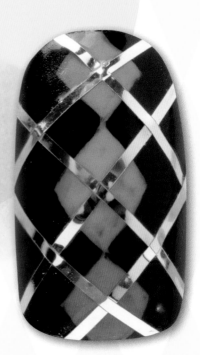

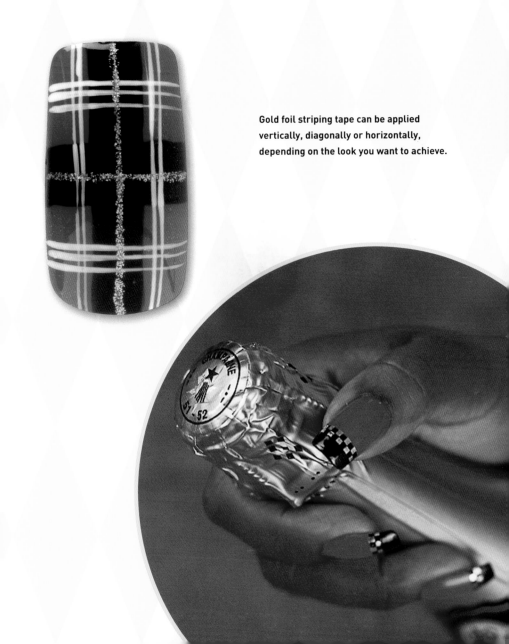

Gold foil striping tape can be applied vertically, diagonally or horizontally, depending on the look you want to achieve.

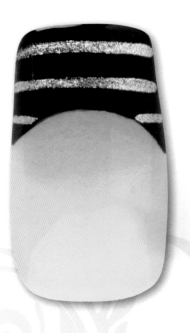
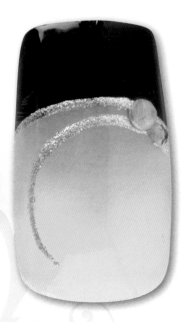

To get perfect curves, take a round sticker and cut it in half. Place the sticker on the nail and paint over it before carefully peeling it away. Other sticker shapes, such as stars and hearts, also make great stencils.

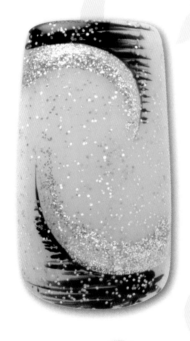
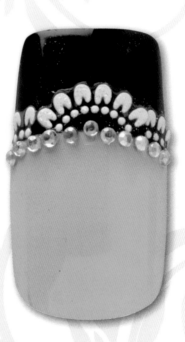

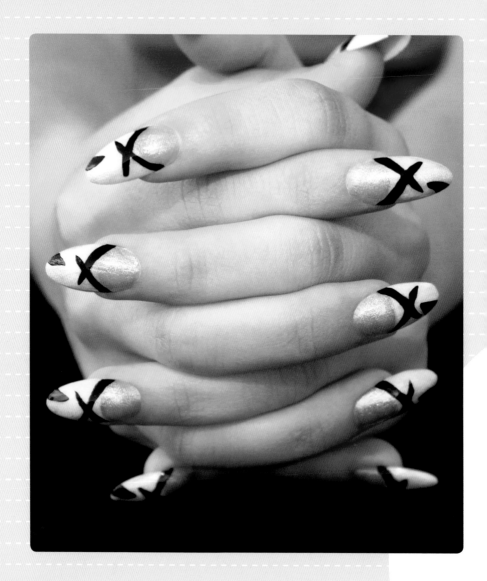

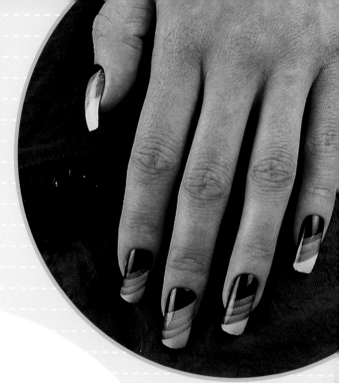

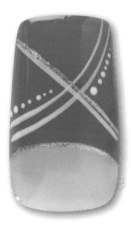

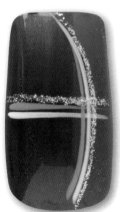

Graduated stripes, like those above, are best achieved in a salon by airbrushing. To recreate the look at home, paint the nail black and then use different dilutions of grey to make progressively lighter stripes.

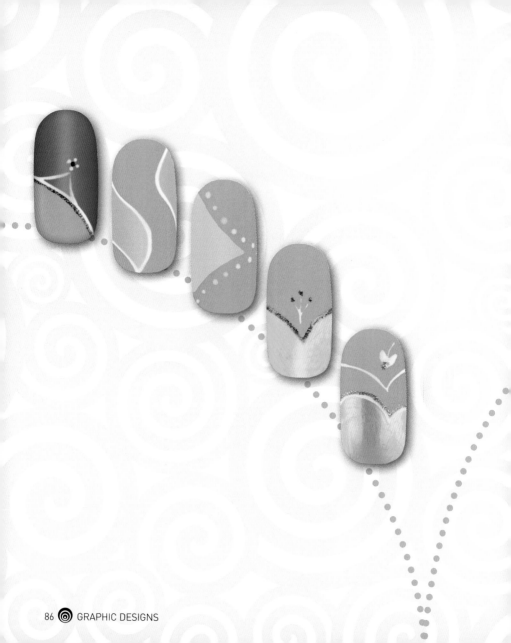

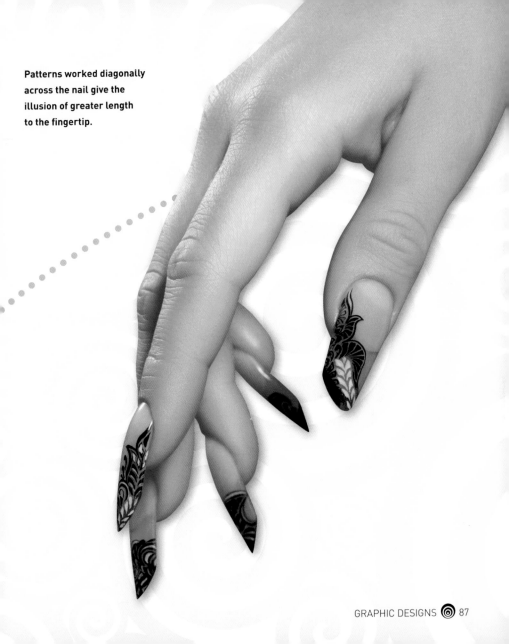

Patterns worked diagonally
across the nail give the
illusion of greater length
to the fingertip.

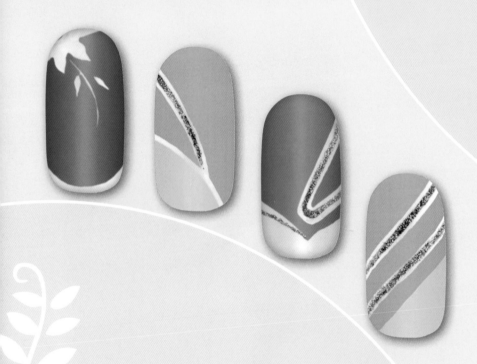

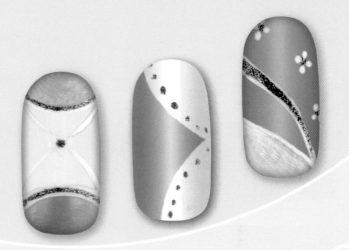

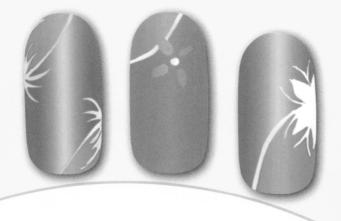

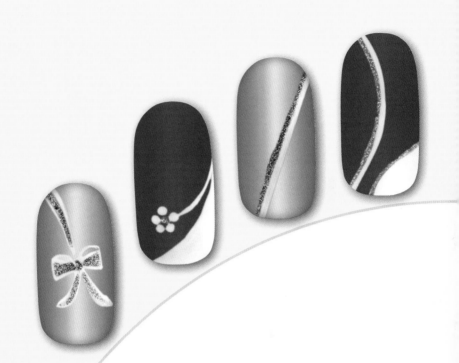

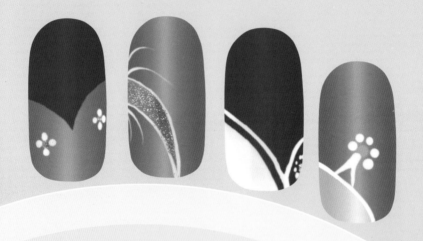

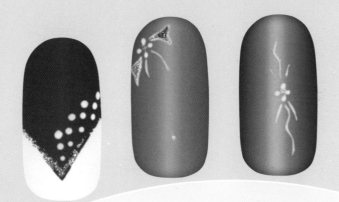

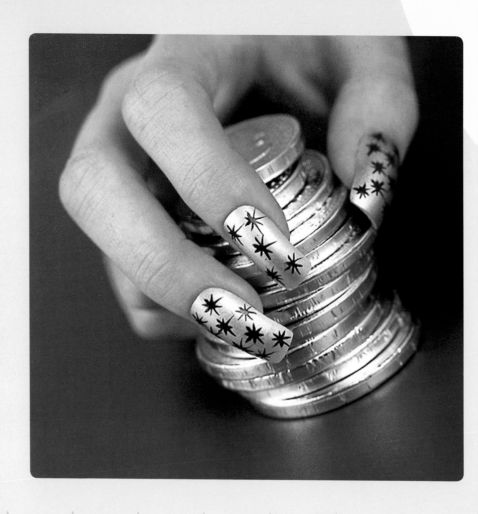

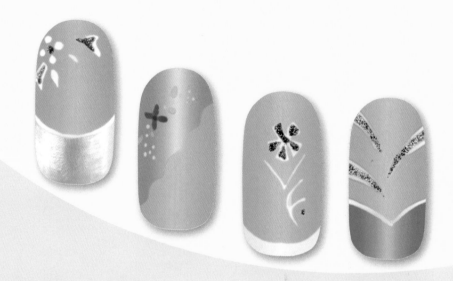

Ordinary silver and glitter nail polishes are often thin and slightly transparent. Choose silver nail paints or metallic polish instead, to create a more dense colour.

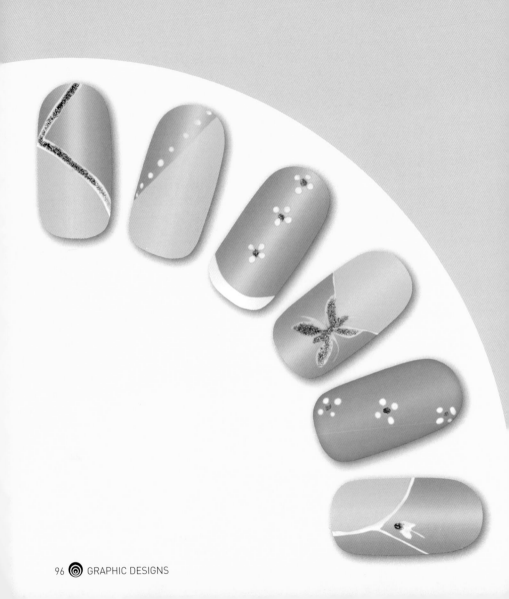

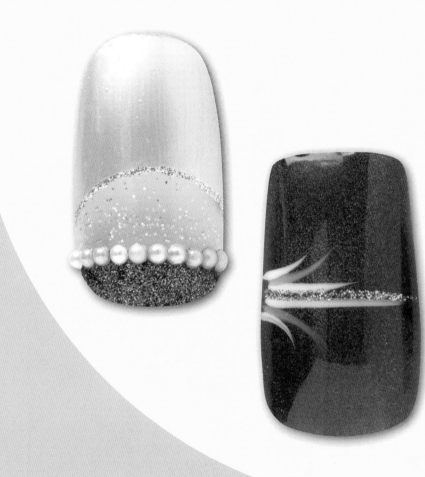

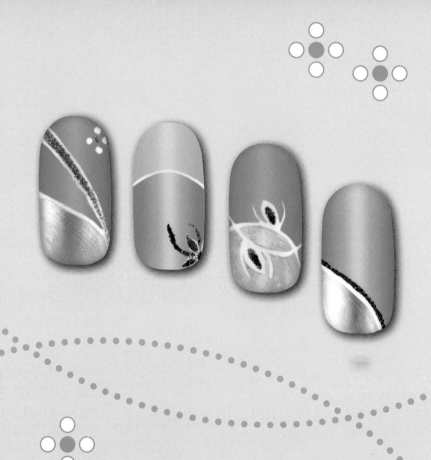

A fan brush was used to create the painterly
effect opposite. Pink then white paint was
feathered across the nail from each side
toward the centre, over a pale blue base coat.

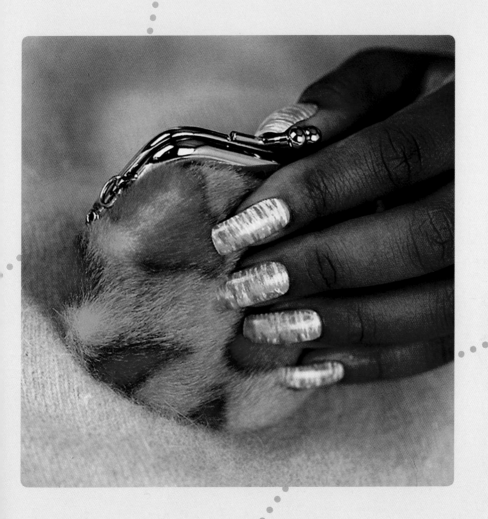

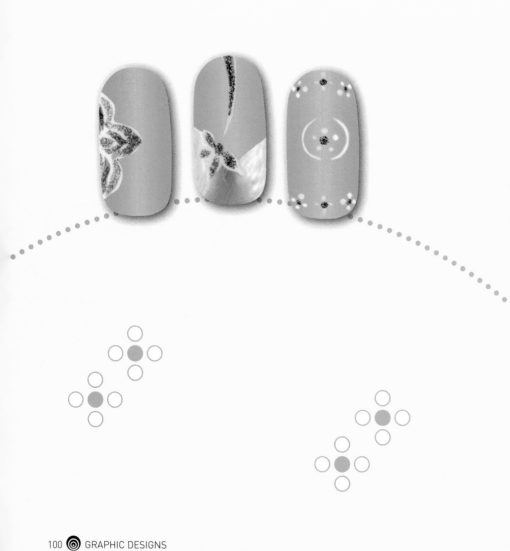

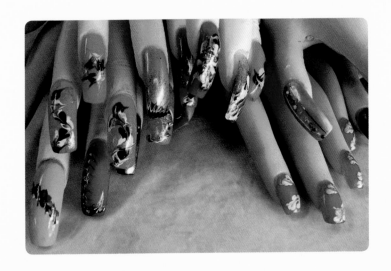

The designs above can be created using marbling. Place several dots of one colour on the nail, then dots of another colour around and on top of the first set of dots. Using a cocktail stick or special-effects tool, swirl the dots together or drag them outward. Try using a criss-cross, S-shaped or figure-eight motion to create different effects.

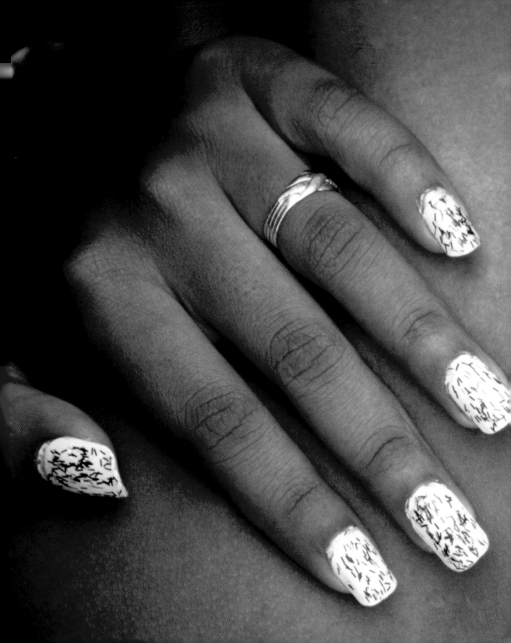

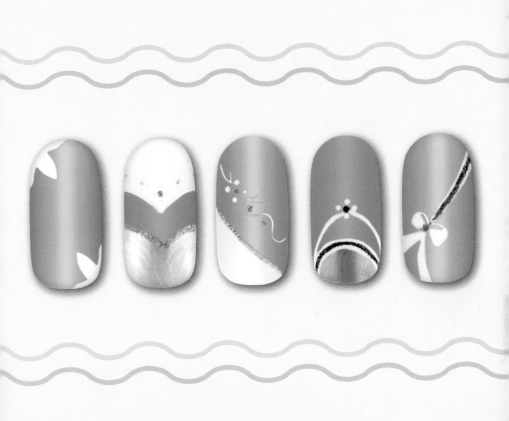

The special effect opposite is achieved by painting a clear, speckled glitter polish over the top of a solid white base colour. For the best impact, choose a bold glitter colour that will show up against the light background.

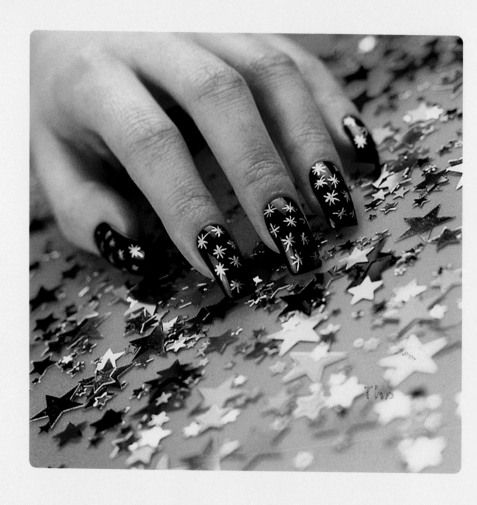

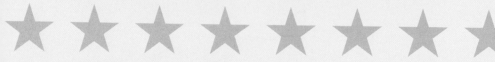

GRAPHIC DESIGNS

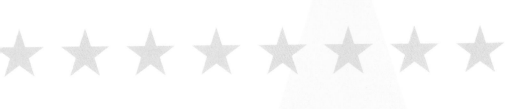

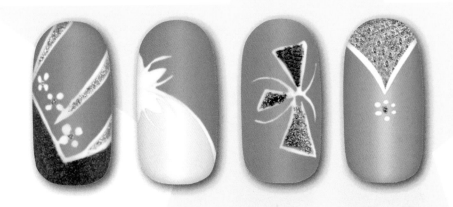

The star design opposite is best achieved with an airbrush or transfer to keep the design uniform. To recreate it, use a stencil to paint a black circle in the centre of the nail then add a star sticker when the paint is dry.

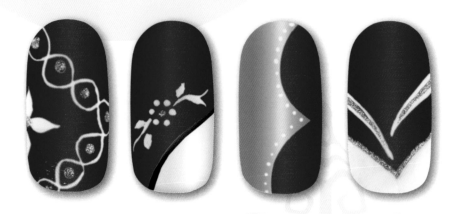

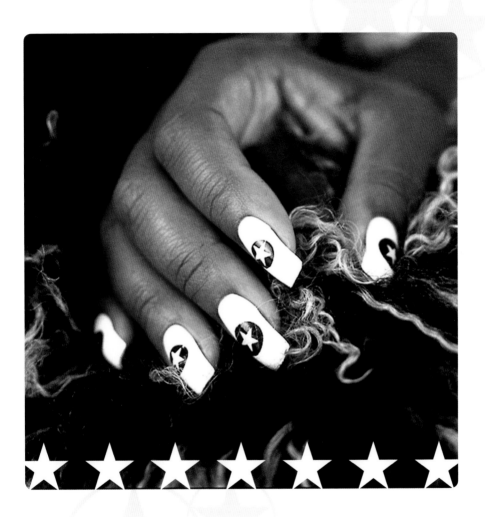

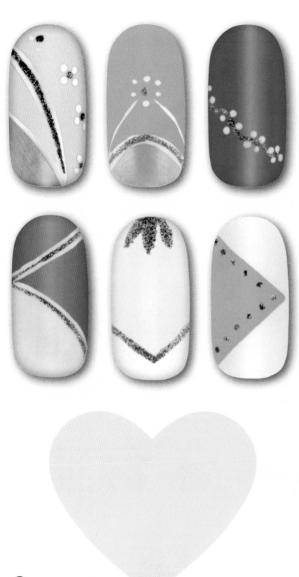

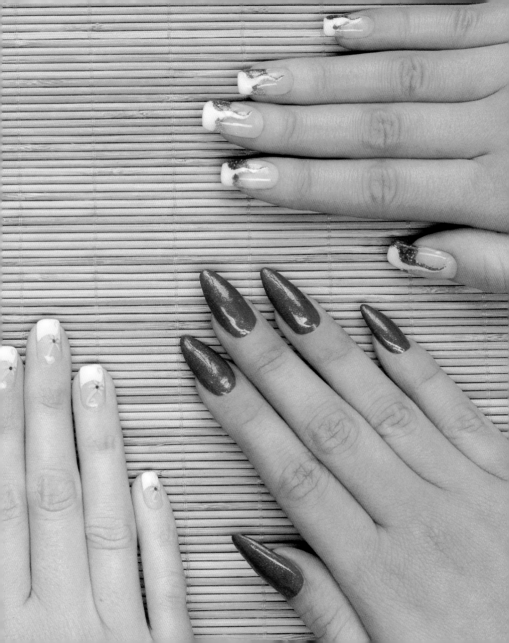

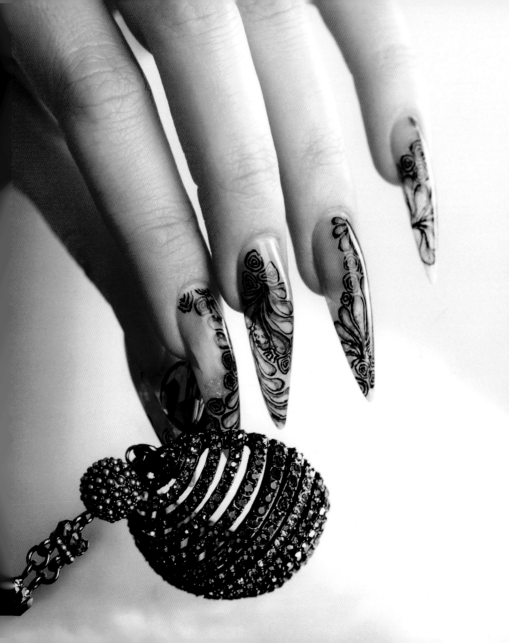

For an intricate, illustrated design, paint
fine black line artwork over a pale pink base
(opposite). If you want to add a hint of sparkle
to the design, paint a little pink glitter over
the top before sealing it.

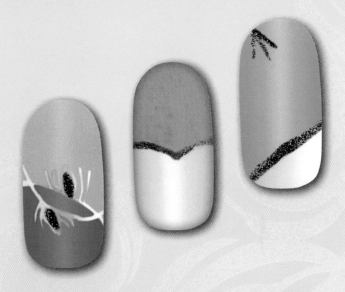

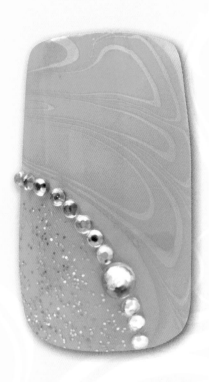

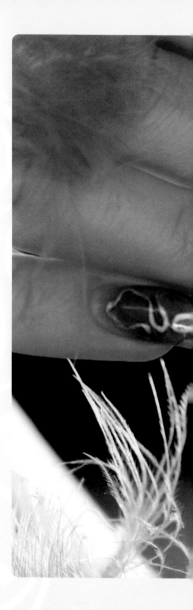

A thick gold outline gives a stained-glass
effect to this design and keeps the jewel-
like colours clearly defined.

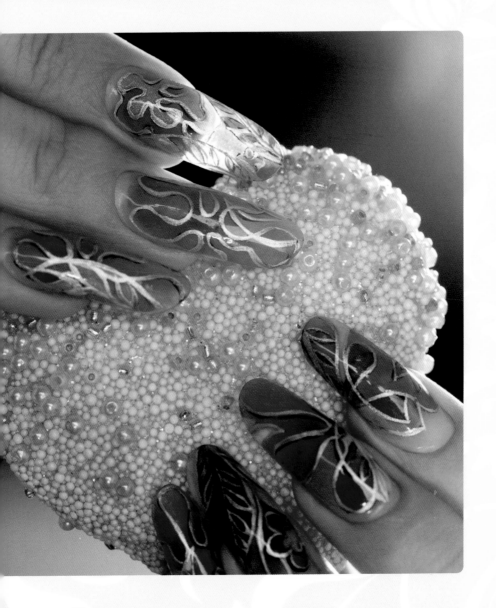

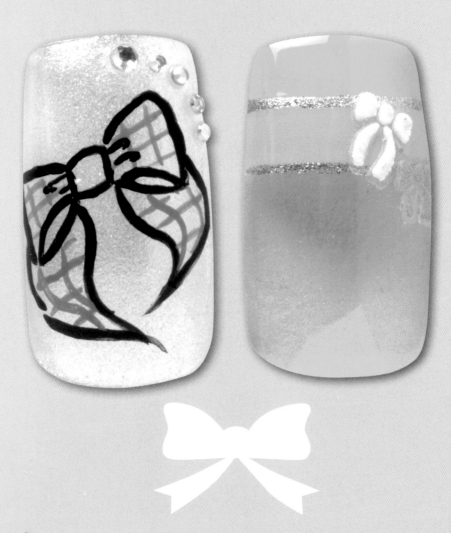

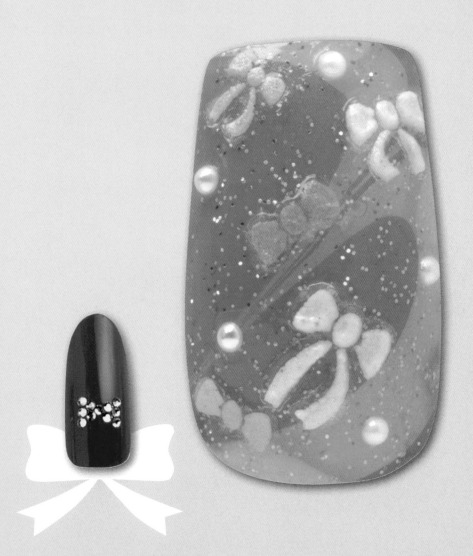

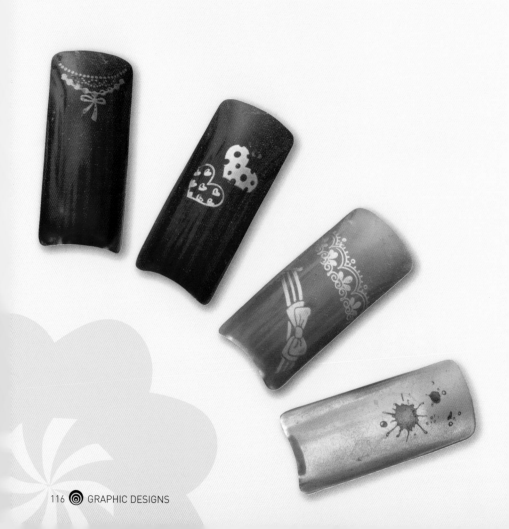

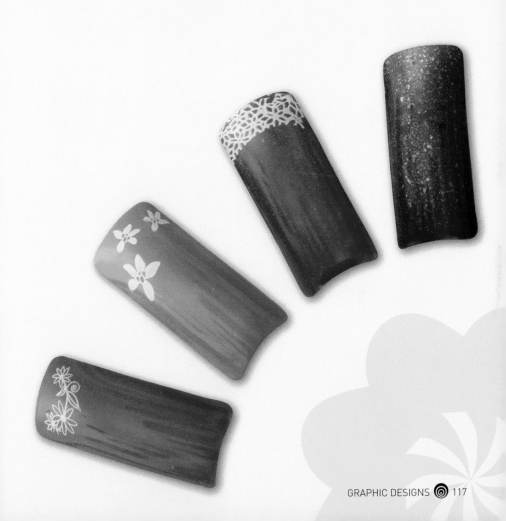

Pictures & Themes

Many people enjoy matching their nail art to a special event, hobby, sports team, music band, holiday or celebration, while others like to paint natural scenes from wildlife, the beach or snowscapes. Transfers are an easy way to add whole pictures to your nails, but if you're good at handpainting, you can create landscapes or skylines, such as the Manhattan skyline, that work across all five fingers. You could also paint portraits, such as celebrity faces, or travel landmarks, such as the Eiffel Tower or Statue of Liberty. National flags, Oriental and Asian themes and lettering, astrological signs, good luck symbols and fantasy figures like dragons and fairies also work well. Animal and nature motifs, such as birds, fish, insects, butterflies, puppies and teddies, can be as delicate and elegant, or as cute and kitsch, as you like.

Cartoon or comic characters – Hello Kitty and Spongebob are favourites the world over – make entertaining designs, as do candles, balloons or cupcakes to honour birthdays. Santas, snowmen, Christmas trees and fairy lights work well for Christmas, and ducks or bunnies are good at Easter (see pages 240–9 for ideas). With all picture designs, you need to be extra careful to work from the largest colour areas first down to the smallest details. Work layer by layer, allowing each coat to dry properly before applying the next.

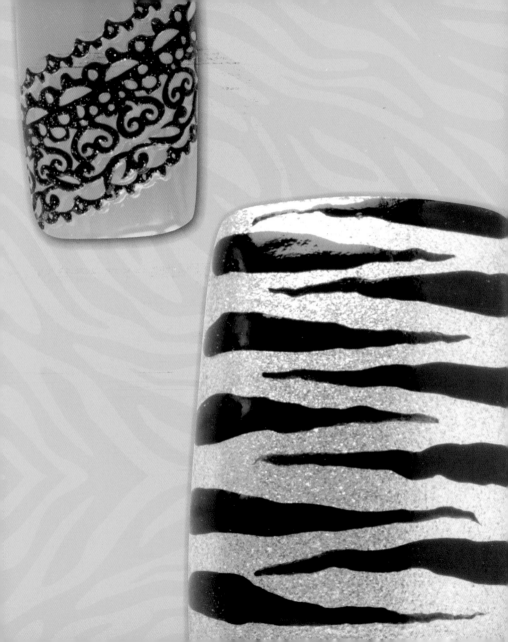

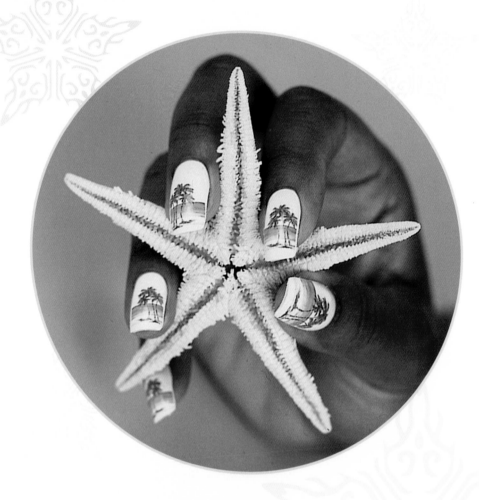

Both the palm tree decoration above and the wave design
opposite were achieved using nail transfers. As with all nail art,
always apply several coats of clear protective sealer on top.

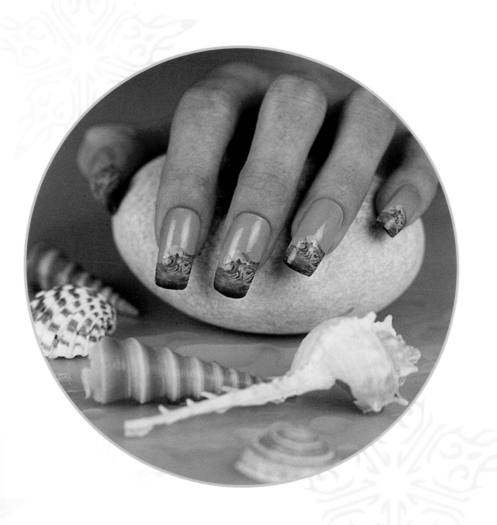

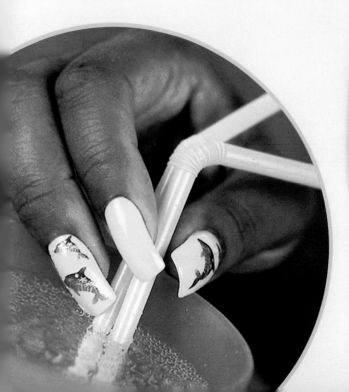

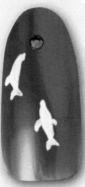

Stick-on stars and gemstones can become part of the picture rather than just embellishment, as with this red stone ball in this dolphin picture, above.

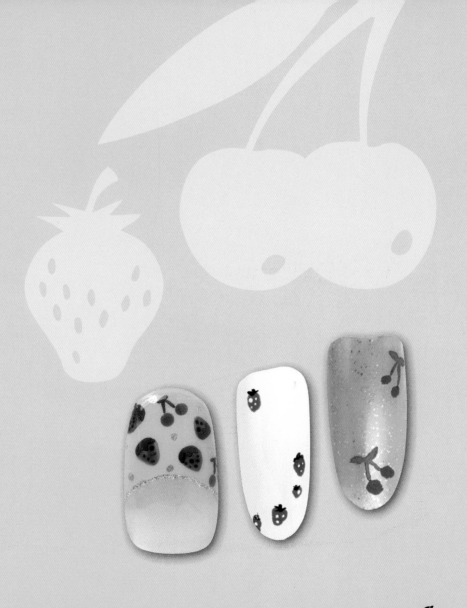

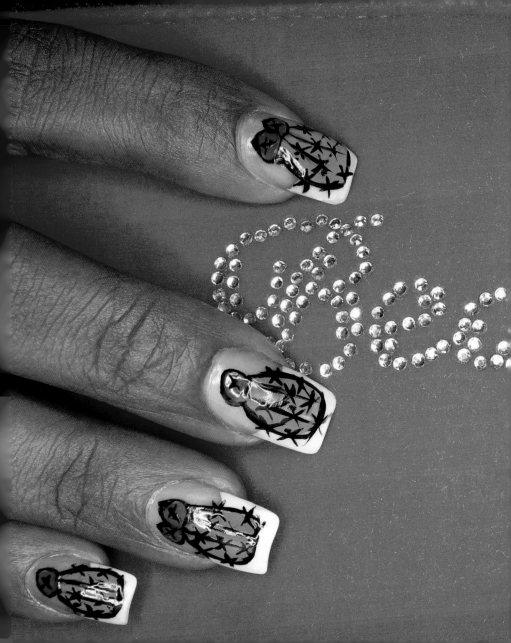

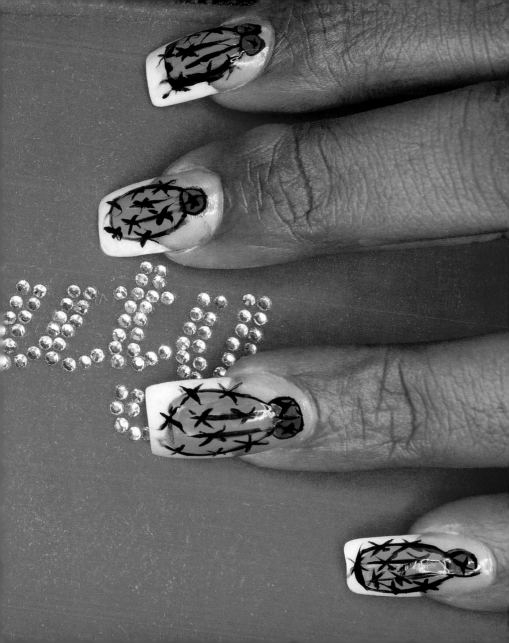

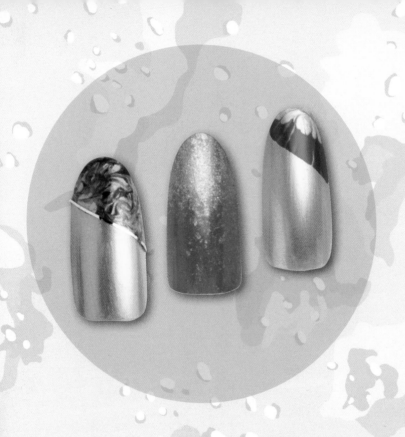

Irregular, squiggly, orange shapes form a camouflage design on a gold background opposite. Black and white details have been added with a fine brush.

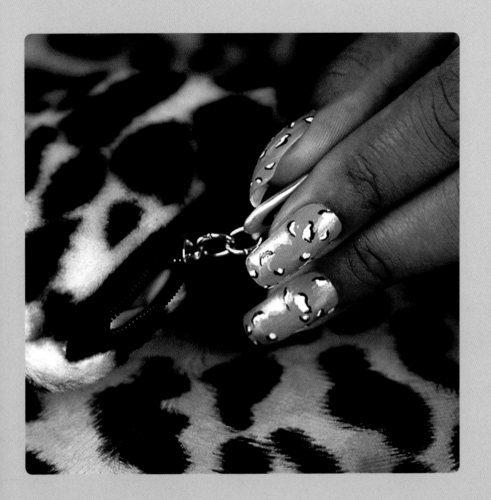

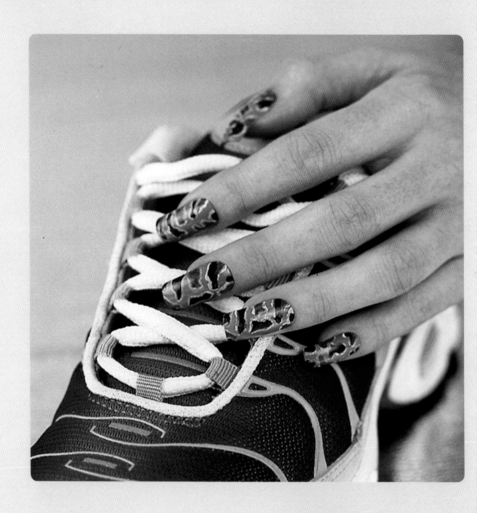

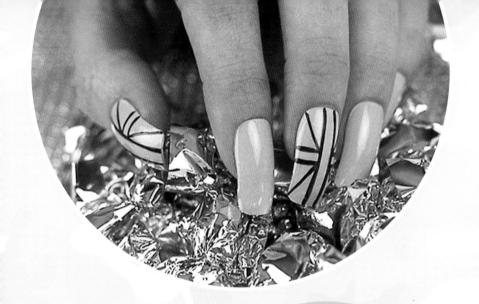

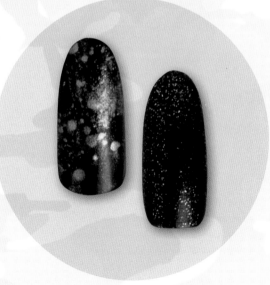

For the camouflage design opposite you may find it easiest to draw the outlines of the shapes first, before filling them in with different shades of blue.

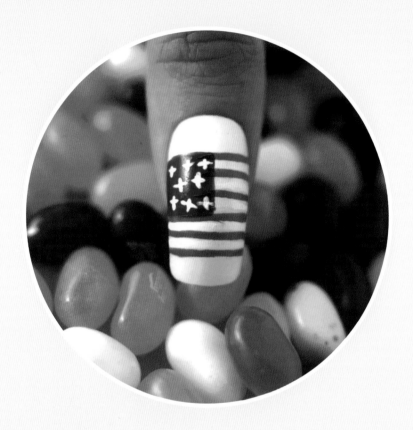

National flags, like the USA's Stars and
Stripes and the UK's Union Jack, are popular
patriotic choices. Alternatively choose your
favourite sports' team's logo or colours.

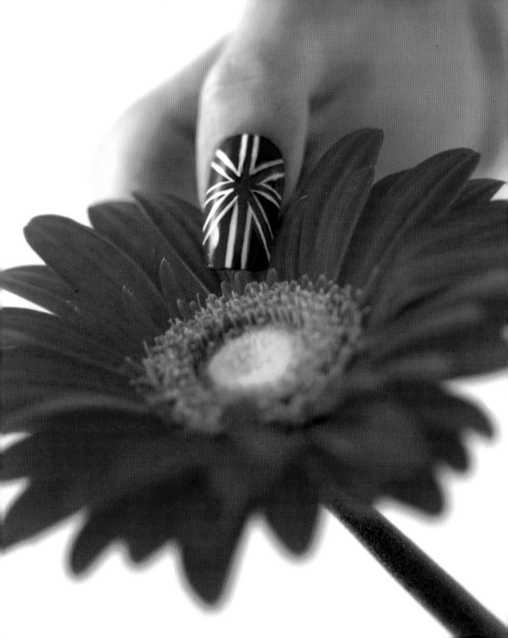

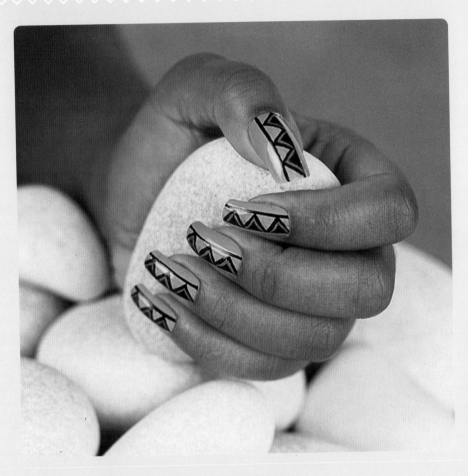

Tribal designs offer great potential for geometric patterning.
Mix up triangles, zigzags and squares, or research Celtic
knotwork and African patterns for ideas.

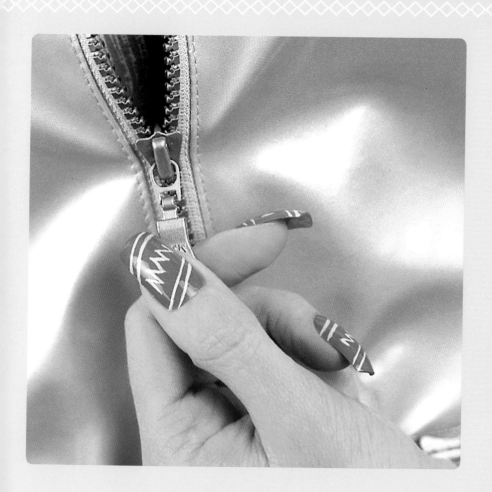

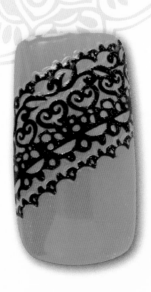
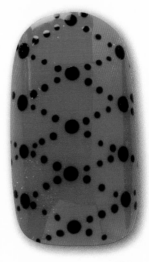
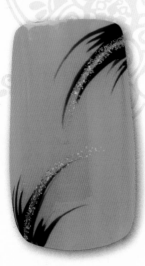

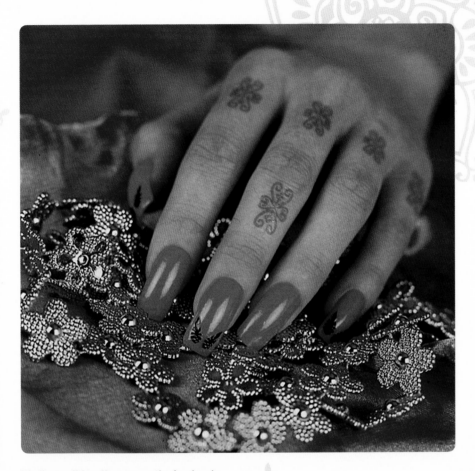

Bindis, traditionally worn on the forehead in parts of Asia, make easy sticker art for nails. They can look especially good for bridal makeup.

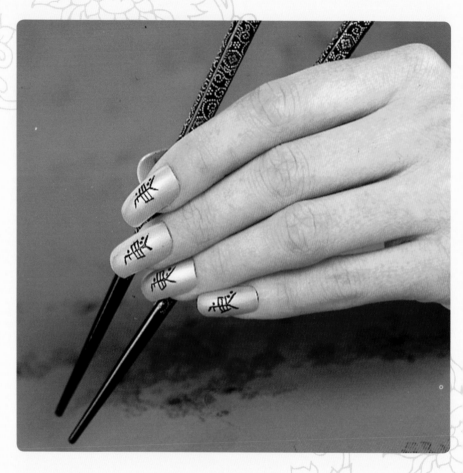

Chinese calligraphy can add an Oriental touch to your designs.
Practise painting the Chinese character of your choice first
before painting it onto your nails. Alternatively, use transfers.

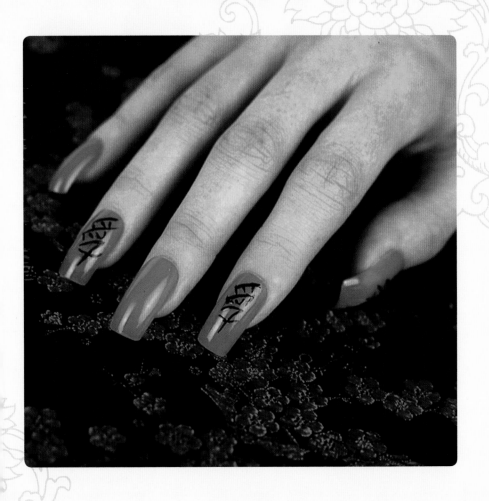

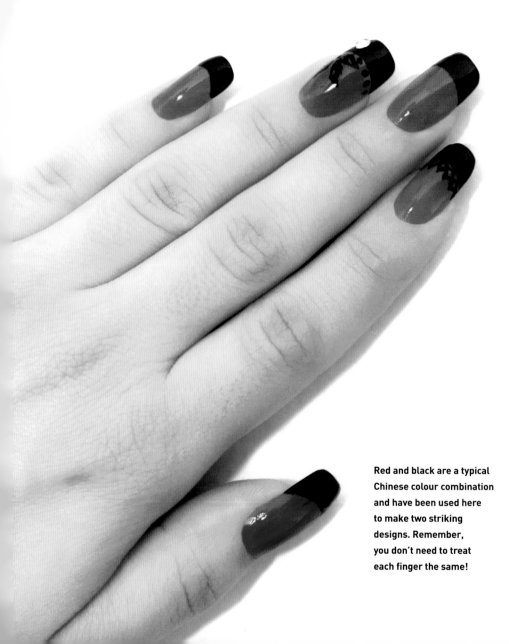

Red and black are a typical
Chinese colour combination
and have been used here
to make two striking
designs. Remember,
you don't need to treat
each finger the same!

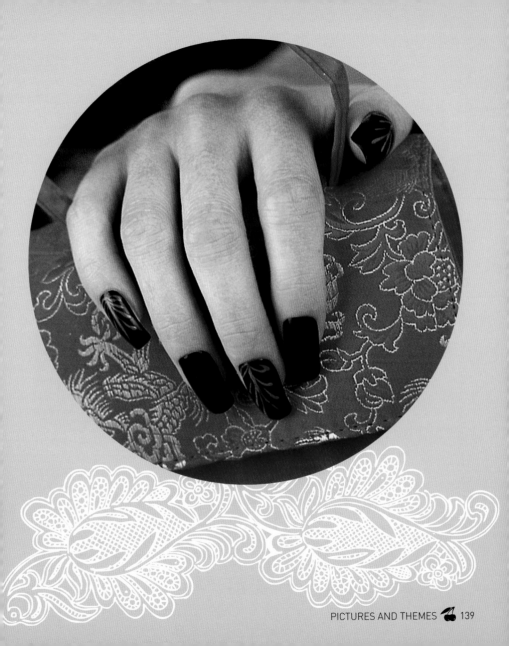

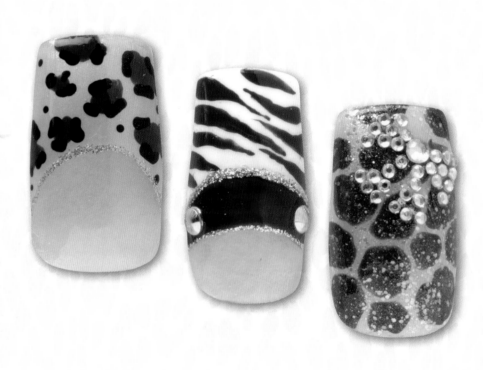

Animal prints can be combined with all sorts of treatments, including glitter and jewels (above). Even a simple design, such as the black nails with gold central stripes opposite, can make a bold statement.

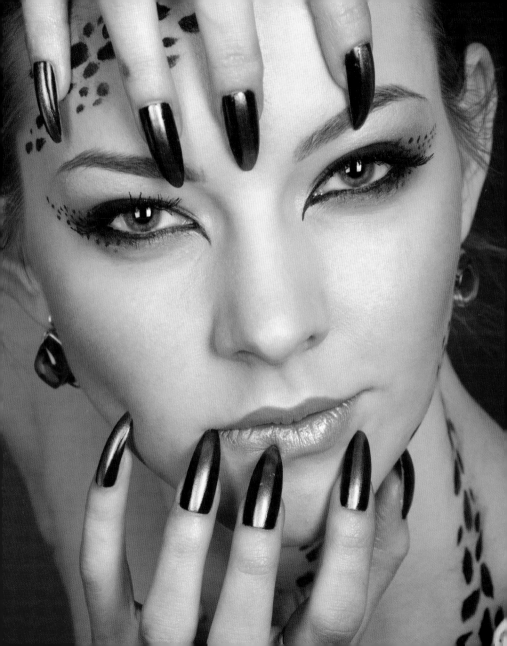

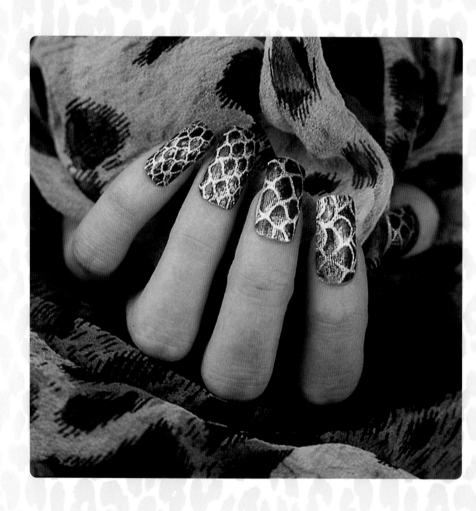

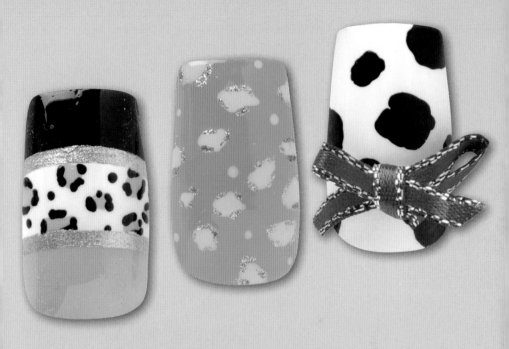

The snakeskin design opposite was made
by using "wraps" – ready-made patterns
that come as stick-on sheets – trimmed
to size. Always ensure you apply the wrap
smoothly to avoid air bubbles.

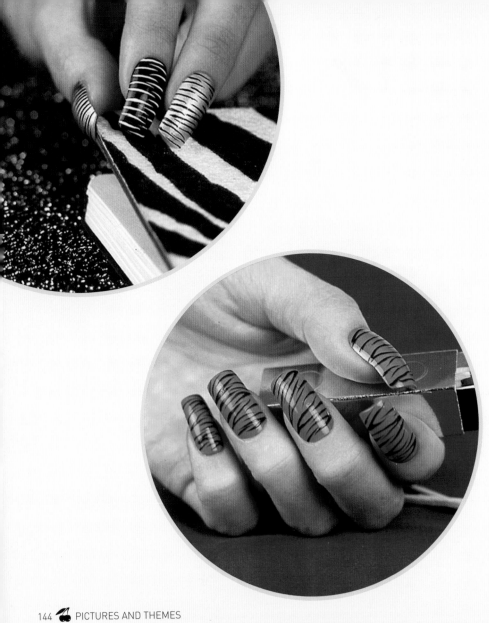

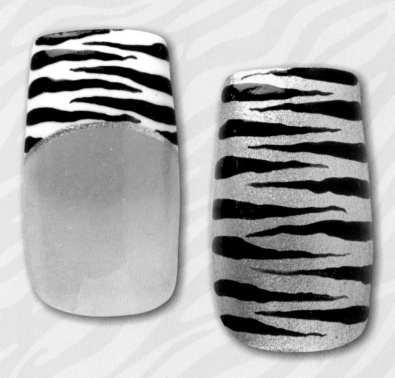

Zebra stripes are some of the most versatile and popular designs, as they are easy for beginners to create. Simply work the stripes from each side toward the centre, making them thicker at the edge. Vary their widths and lengths too.

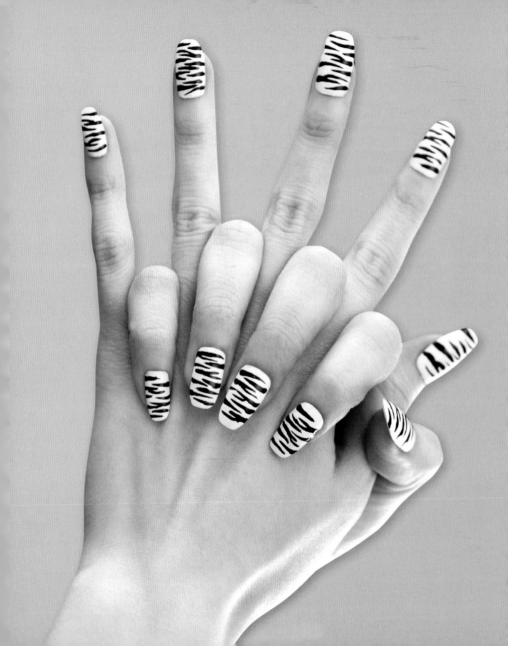

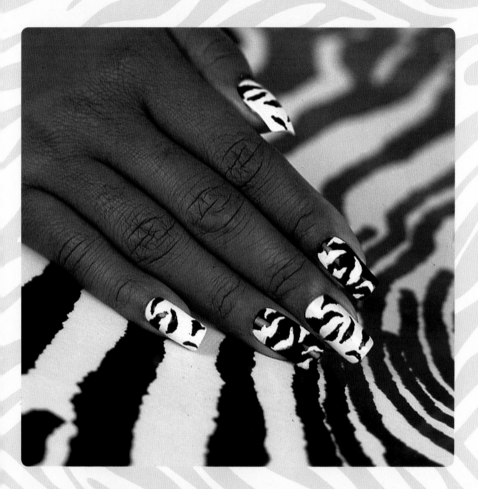

Use more random shapes to create the black-and-white tiger stripe above – you could also re-create the design in traditional, tiger-coloured browns and golds.

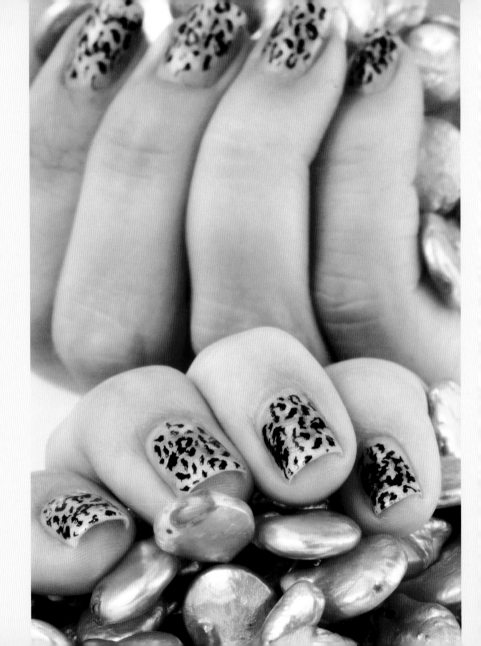

For a unique effect, create your animal prints in a variety of different colours. You could also paint black spots on top of a multicoloured background (opposite).

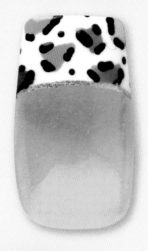

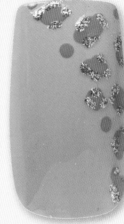

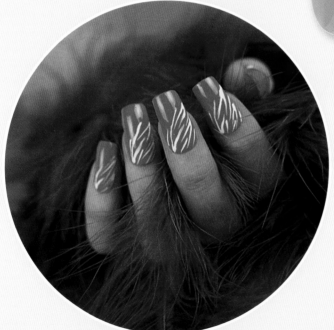

Glitter & Metallic

Glitter, metallic and chrome paints, and crackle glaze, can also be used to create a range of special effects. Glitter and metallics can be used to enhance details of the design, form a background shimmer as part or all of the base colour, or be densely layered over the whole nail or just at the tip. For a "sprinkle" effect, you can make the glitter very thick and concentrated at the tip and lighter through the rest of the nail – an easy way to do this is to use a sponge to build up thin layers. Alternatively, pour loose glitter into a small cup, paint your nail on just the tip and dip the wet polish into the glitter. Blow excess glitter away and allow to dry the nail.

Different colours of glitter can be blended together, layered on top of each other, or painted on in stripes. Because glitters are available in so many colours, and in everything from dust particles and flakes to tiny sparkles, confetti, stars, hearts and other shapes, there are endless ways to use it. Some glitters provide only a subtle shimmer, so you may want to add extra loose glitter powder to the gel or polish to achieve better coverage.

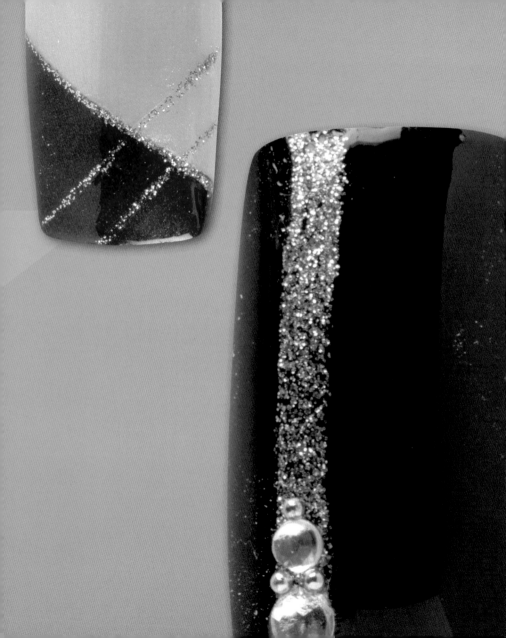

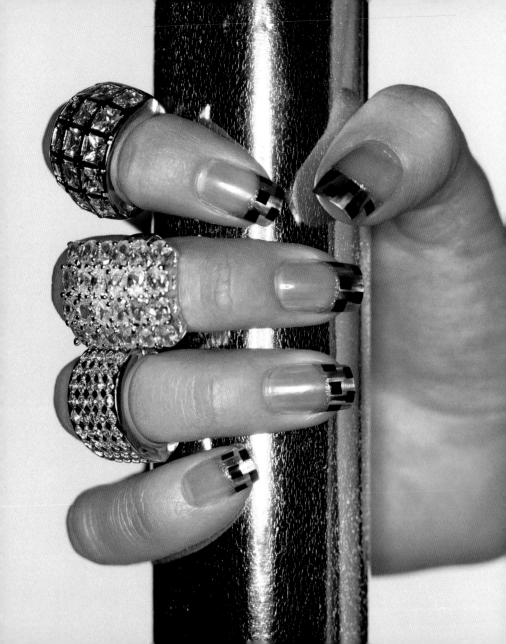

Foil strips can be used to replicate a glitter or metallic painted effect. When using strips, it is often useful to glue a diamanté, stud or pearl on the strip to help anchor it.

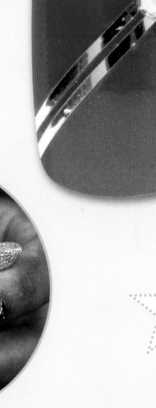

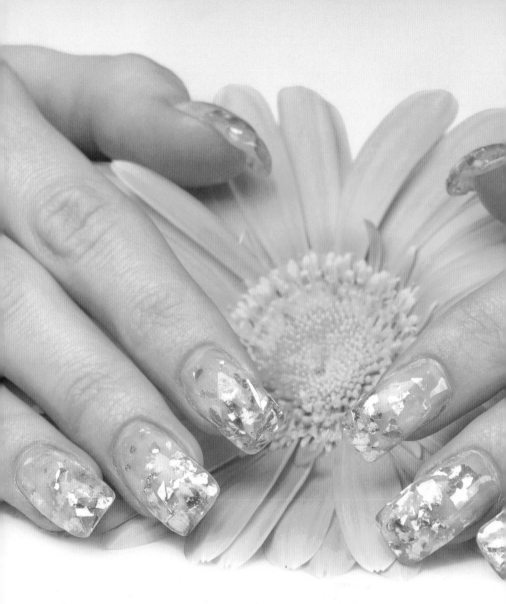

Clear nail polishes with sparkly shapes and
particles incorporated in them have been
used to create these two designs.

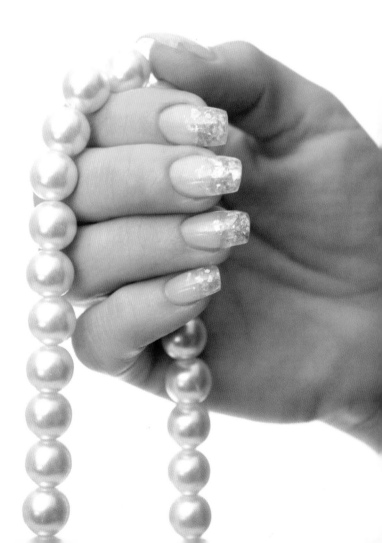

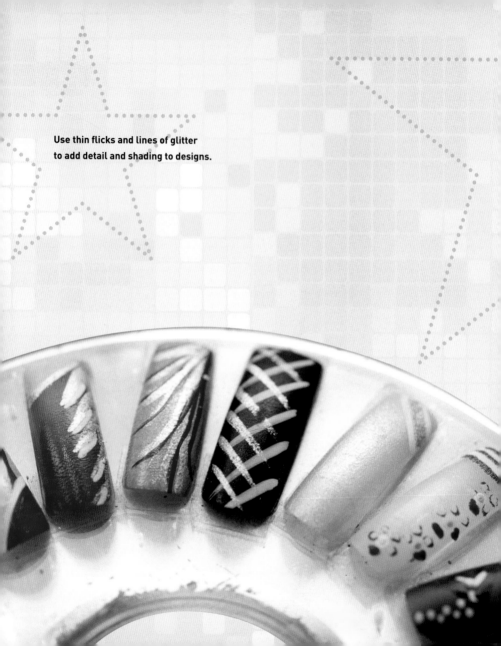

Use thin flicks and lines of glitter
to add detail and shading to designs.

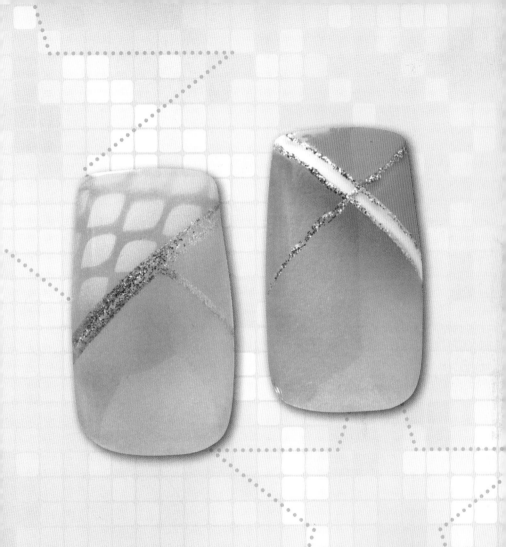

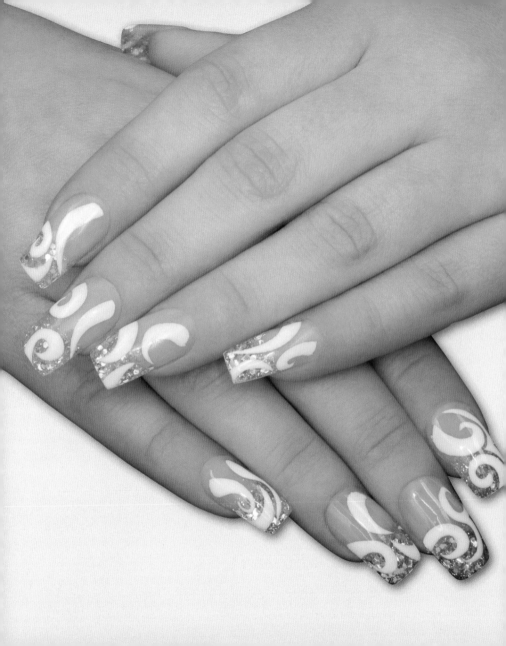

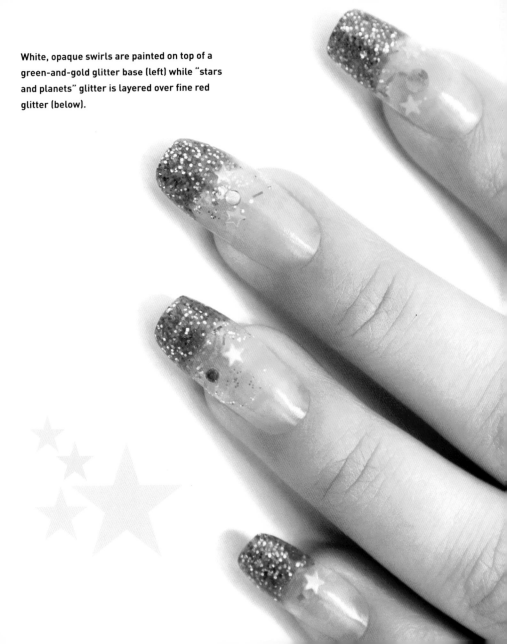

White, opaque swirls are painted on top of a green-and-gold glitter base (left) while "stars and planets" glitter is layered over fine red glitter (below).

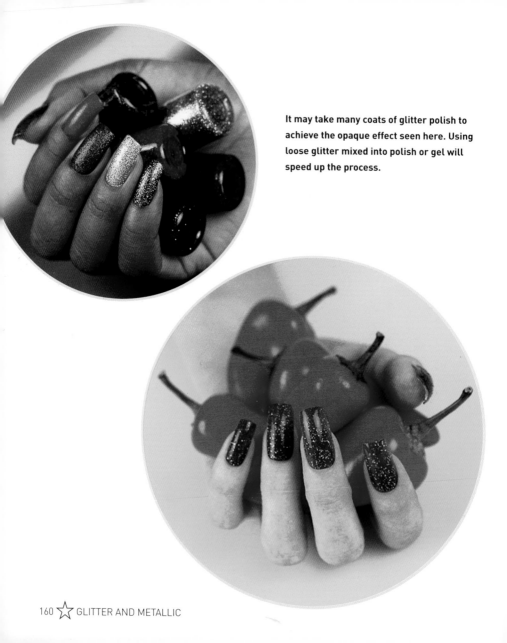

It may take many coats of glitter polish to achieve the opaque effect seen here. Using loose glitter mixed into polish or gel will speed up the process.

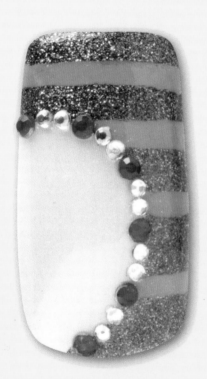
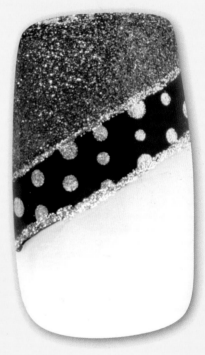

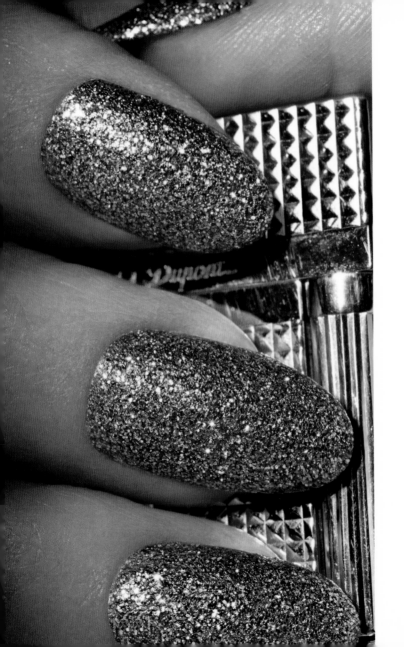

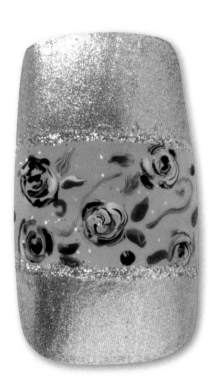
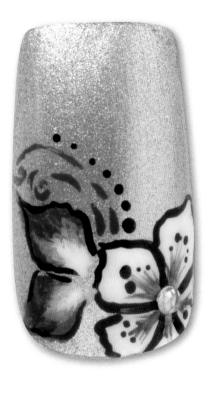

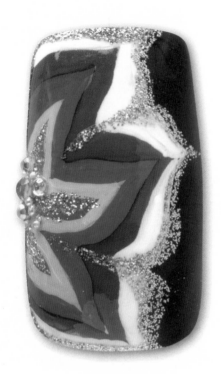
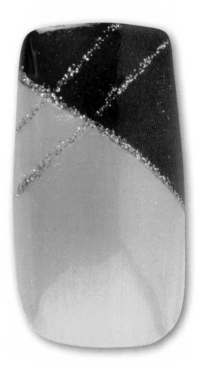

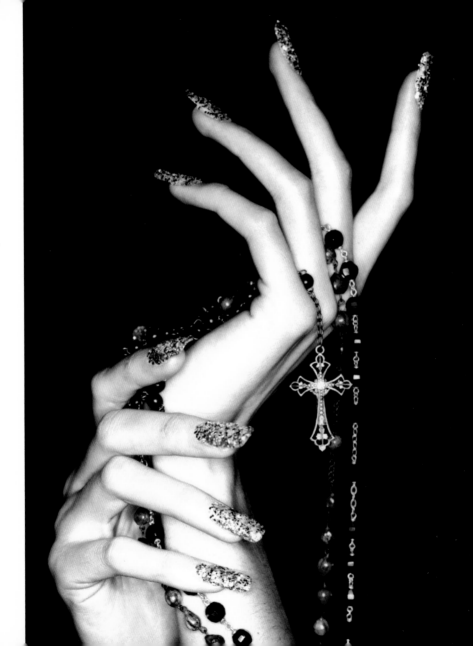

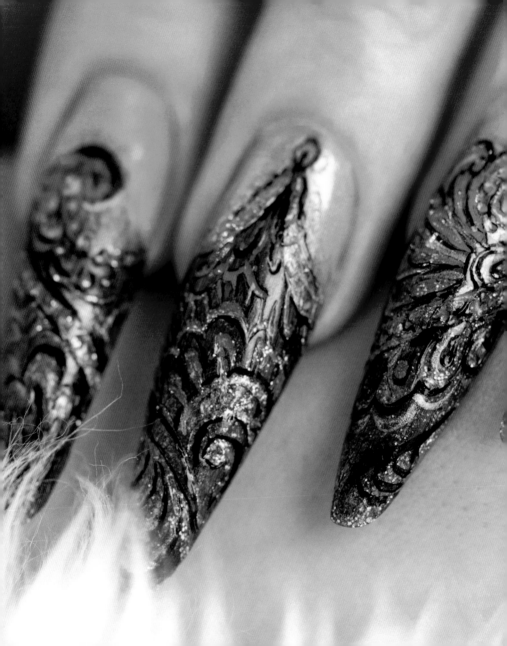

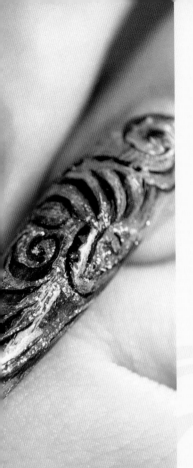

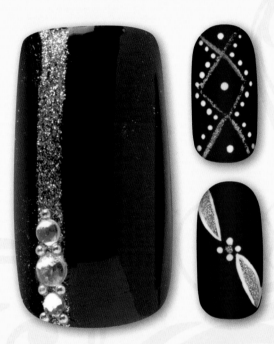

Layers of gold glitter were worked with fine black linework to create this intricate effect. A deep brown/gold was used as the base (and more densely applied at the tips), while a lighter gold tone was used to highlight aspects of the design.

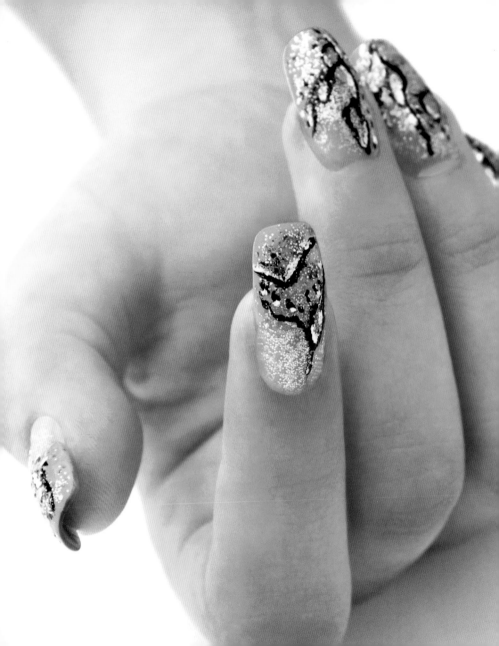

For the glitter camouflage design below, first create the irregular shapes by outlining them in white paint. Fill in each area with a different glitter colour and finish by tracing over the white outlines in black.

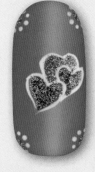
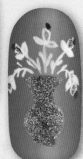

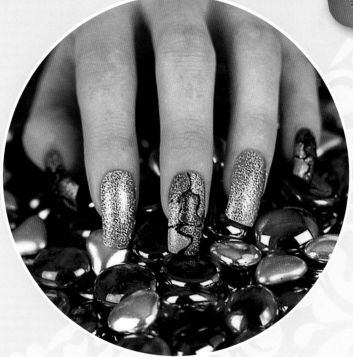

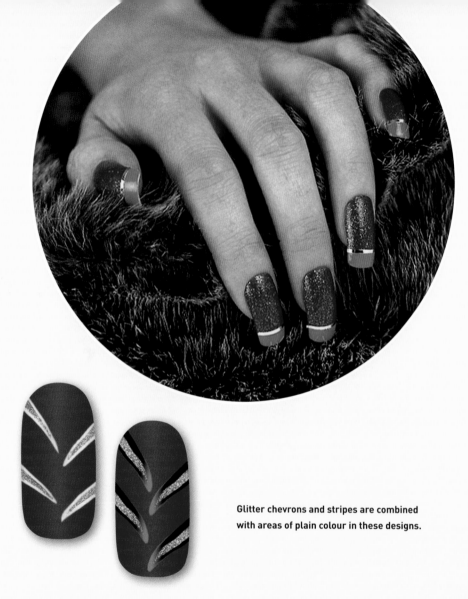

Glitter chevrons and stripes are combined
with areas of plain colour in these designs.

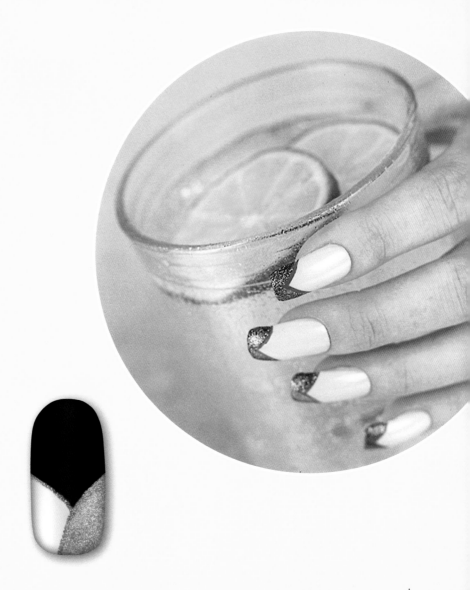

Jewelled Designs

Gemstones, diamantés, pearls, jewelled strips and bindis are all available for creating jewelled nail art designs. To apply, use tweezers or a special applicator to dip the jewel or stone into a drop of nail gel or nail glue and transfer it onto the nail. A cuticle stick can be useful to help move the jewels into position.

You can buy specially-made jewels and stickers from nail art supply stores, or find your own stones by recycling your old jewellery – make sure the pieces are small and have flat bottoms. You can buy stones shaped like petals, teardrops, diamonds, square-cut, bows, flowers and heart shapes, as well as snowflakes, stars, tiny bullion beads, hologram pieces and metallic studs (perfect for the rock chick look). Body gems or even small stones and studs that are designed for gluing onto clothing can also be incorporated into nail art. Stationery shops may have a range of other useful products, such as confetti shapes and star stickers.

Often it is easiest to think about transforming a normal painted design into a jewelled one by adding small stones. However, if you are ambitious, fairly skilled and patient, you can go for a fully jewel-encrusted look. This can be a bit painstaking and time-consuming, so you might consider doing just one nail.

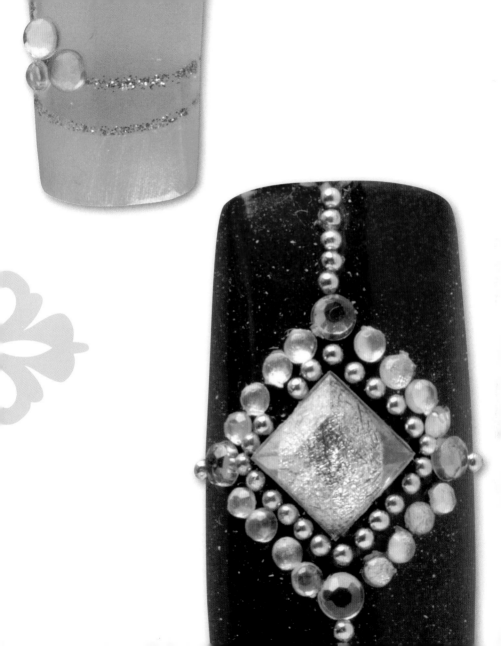

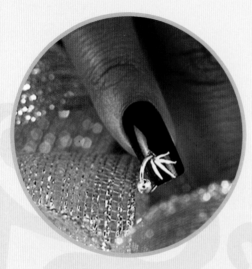

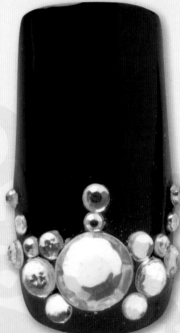

The ultimate in jewelled designs is the pierced nail. This is best done on a false press-on nail and by a professional, but if you do it yourself only ever use a piercing tool designed for this purpose and ensure the nail is coated with several layers of protective base coat. Jewellery hoops can be interchanged to coordinate with your design.

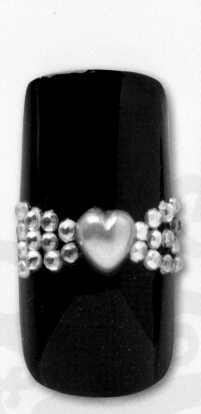
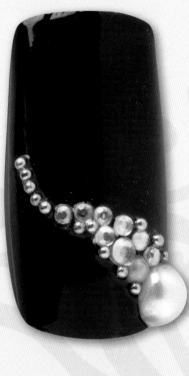

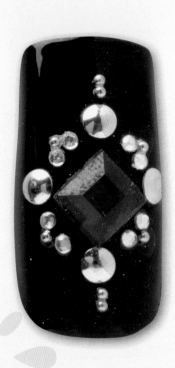
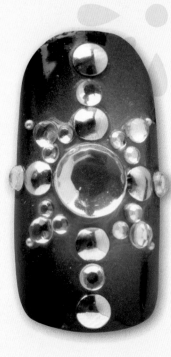

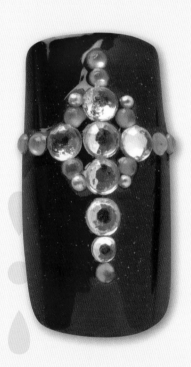
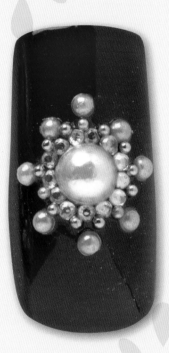

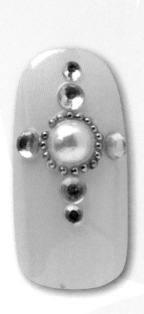
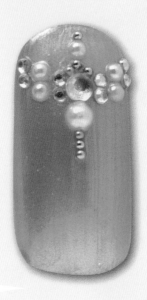
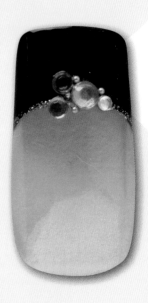

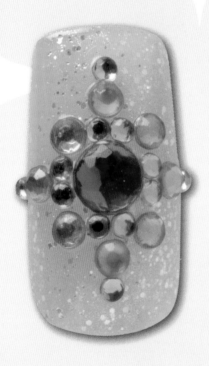
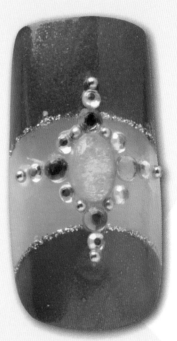

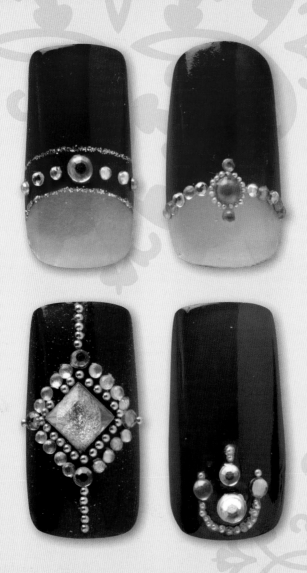

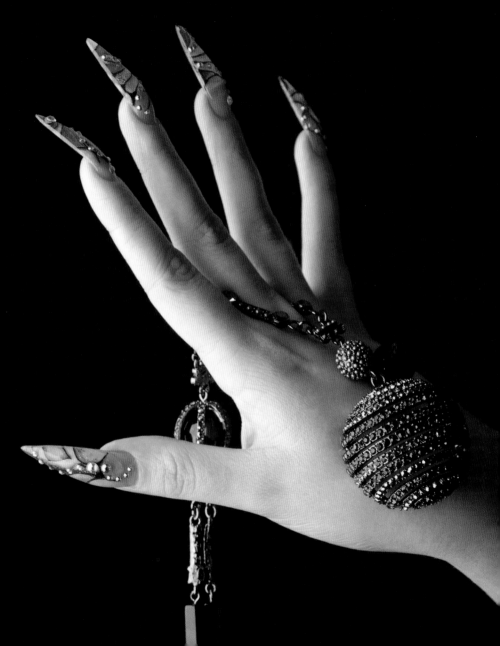

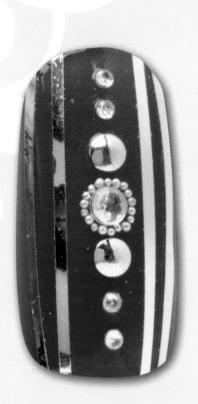
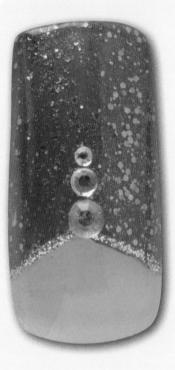

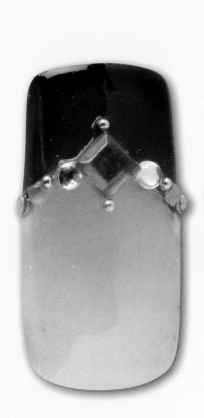
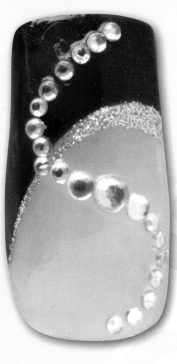

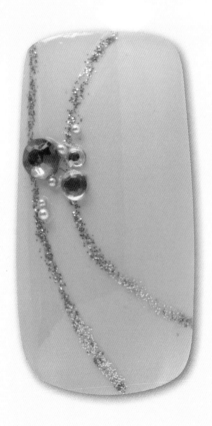
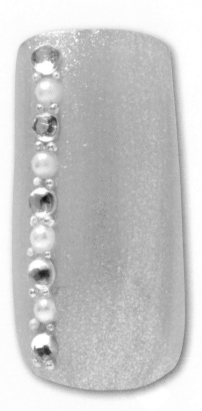

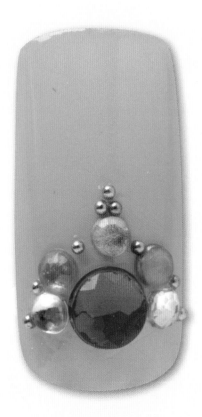
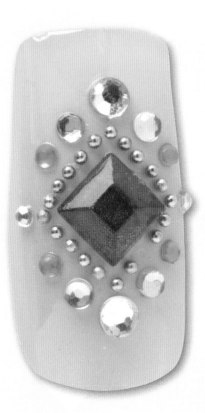

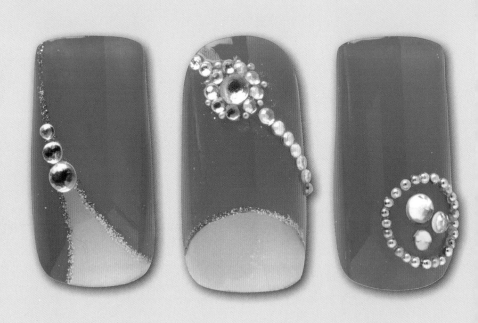

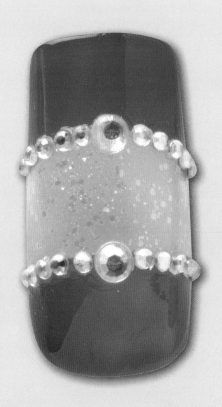
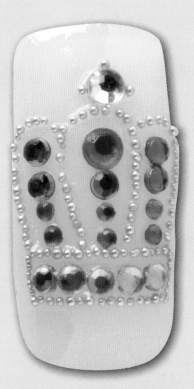

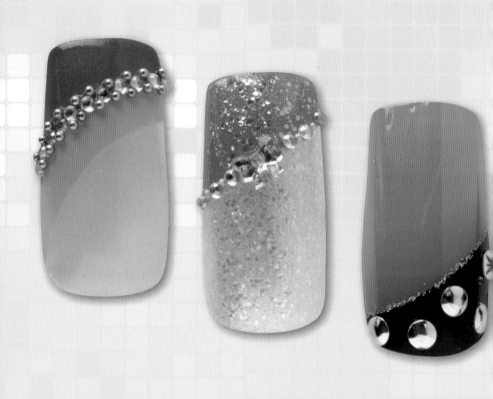

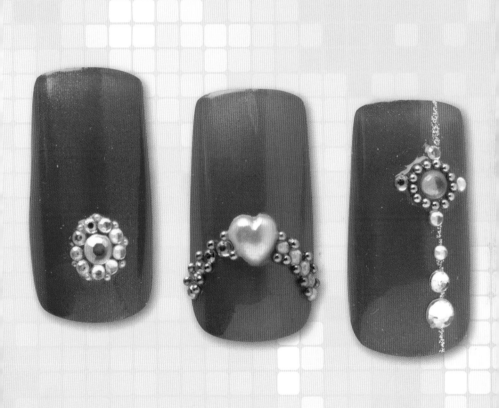

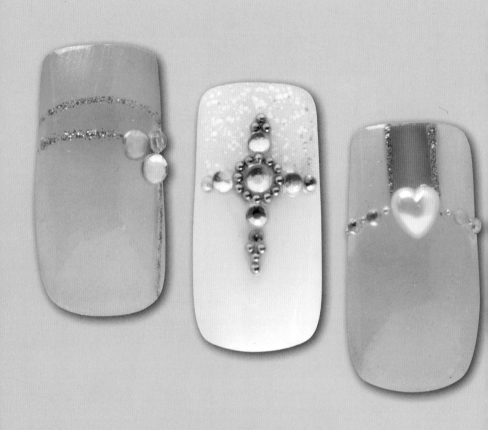

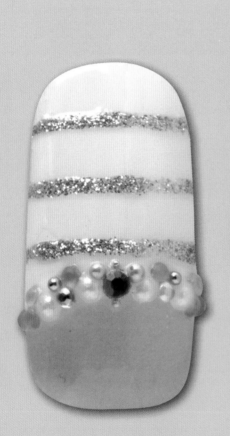
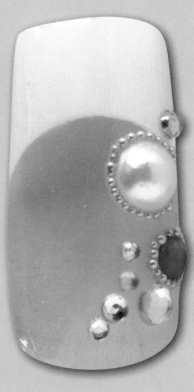

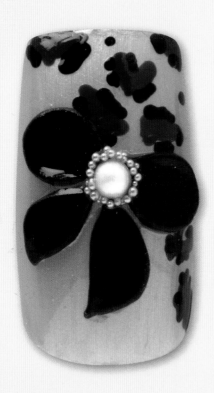
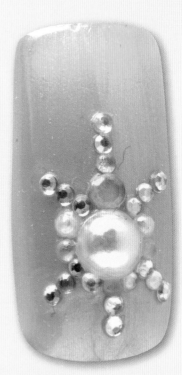

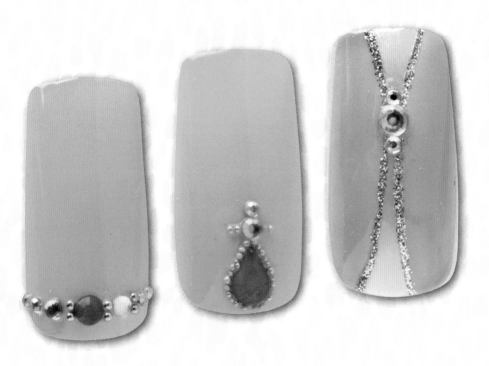

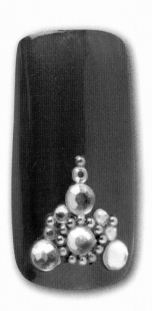
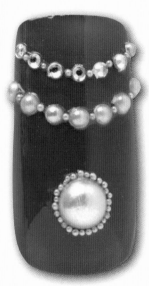
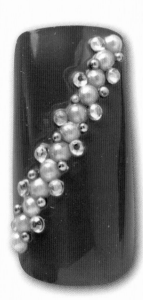

Each nail here has been designed with a different type of sparkling gemstone – round, square-cut, oblong and circular – all stuck onto a blue base.

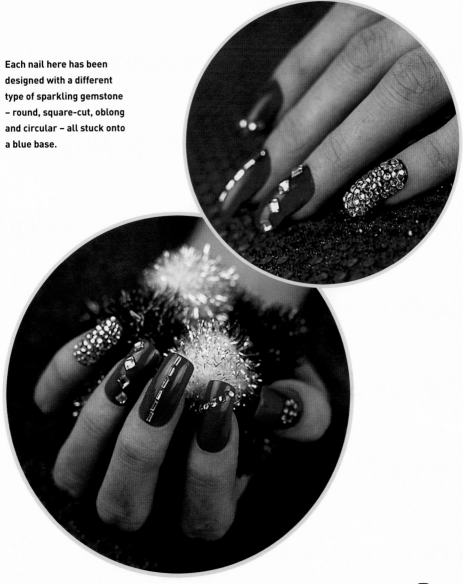

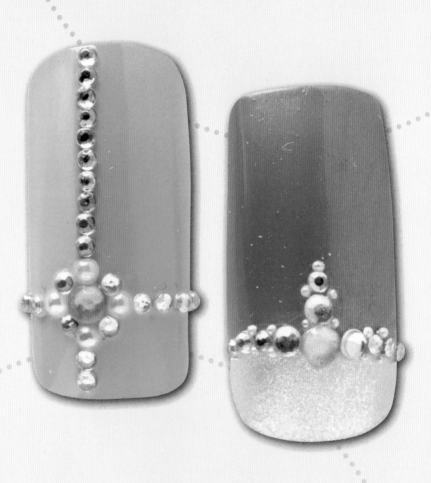

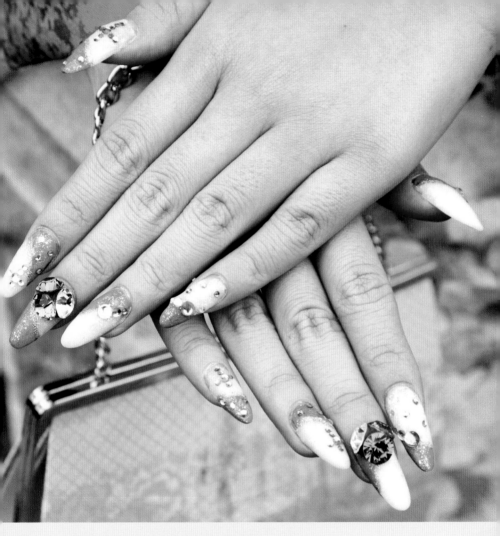

When arranging straight rows of gemstones, simply draw
a thin line of glue and place the stones along it, one by one.
Arrange them closely so that they give each other support.

Romantic & Bridal

All sorts of romantic themes can be created in nail art – visually, in the form of hearts and flowers, by incorporating words such as "love", or by spelling out the name or initials of a loved one. When planning your bridal design, it is always a good idea to draw out your designs on paper and to colour them up before you begin, that way you can experiment with different colourways and compositions before making your final decision. Nail art can take a considerable amount of time, so you may want to plan and organize carefully, especially if you are doing nails for the "big day".

For bridal designs, think of ideas that will work with the wedding plan – flowers, colours and any over-arching theme, such as beach, country, fantasy or garden. Designs can range from relatively plain and simple, which any bride would feel comfortable wearing, to more ornate versions that only the adventurous few might consider. There are nail technicians and salons that specialize in coordinating your nails with your bridal theme, and they can also work with you to get a look for yourself and your entire wedding party.

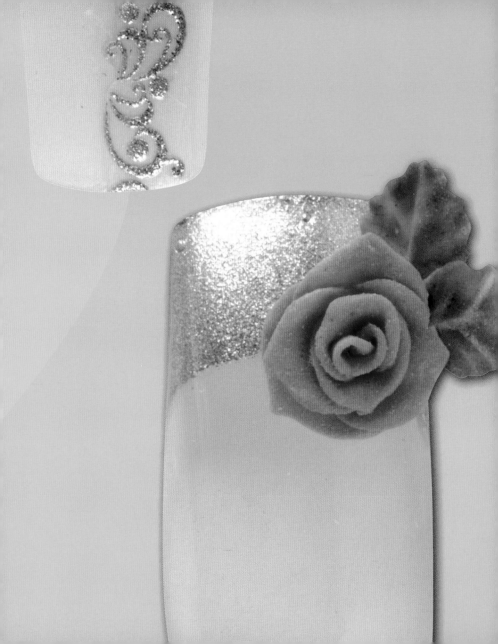

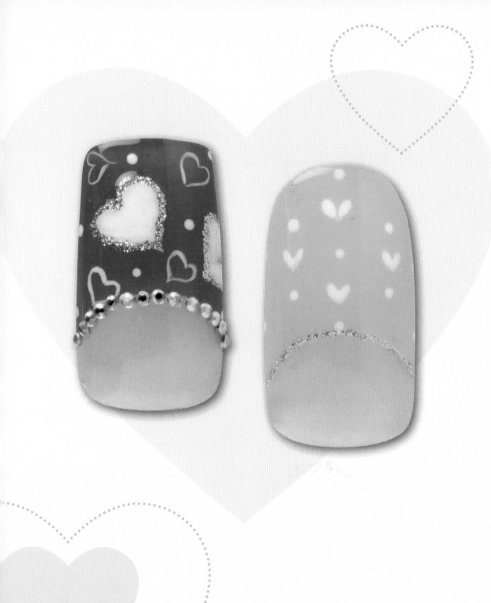

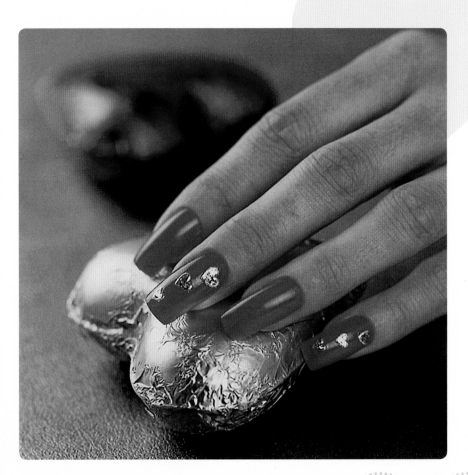

Three foil, stick-on hearts, arranged in a
diagonal line down the centre of red nails
on the thumb, second and fourth fingers,
make a simple but effective bridal look.

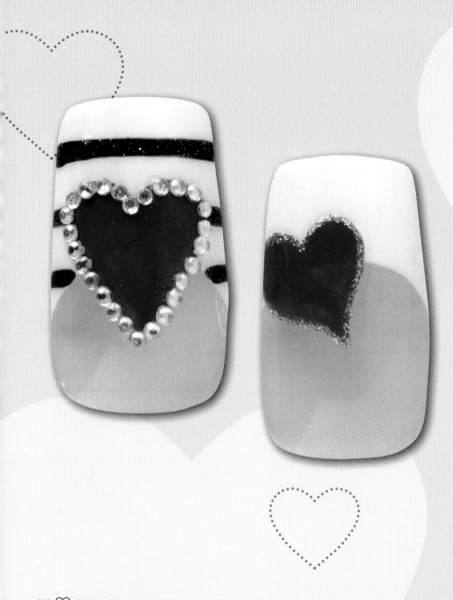

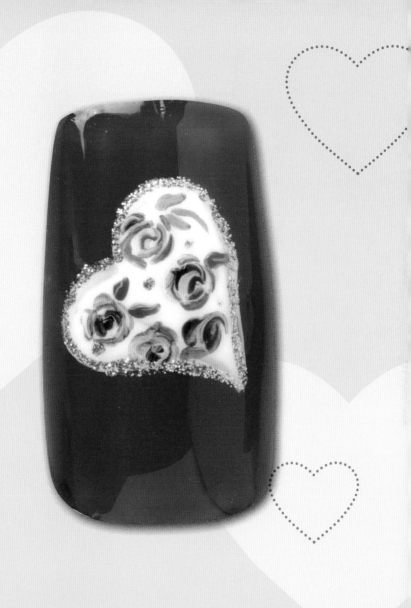

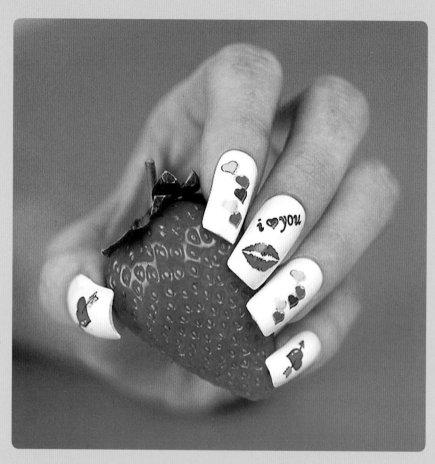

Make a declaration of love with these transfers applied over several coats of white colour. An easy way to create a heart is to join two teardrop shapes together.

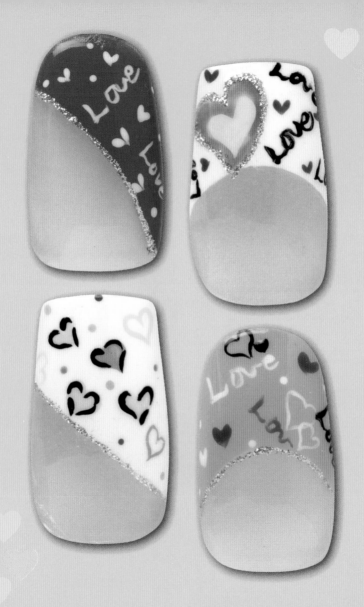

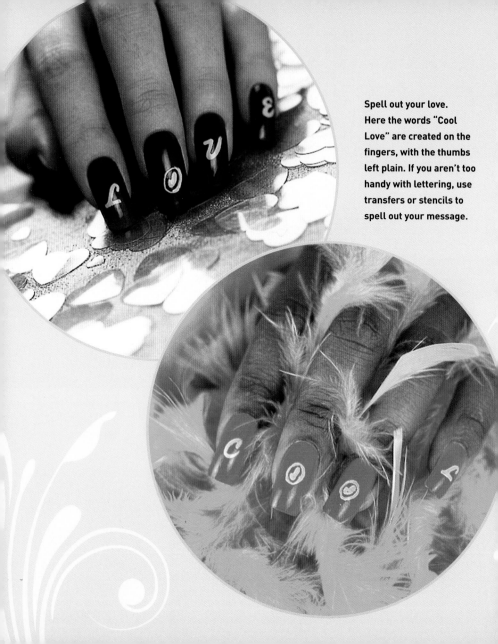

Spell out your love. Here the words "Cool Love" are created on the fingers, with the thumbs left plain. If you aren't too handy with lettering, use transfers or stencils to spell out your message.

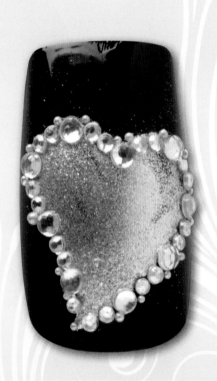
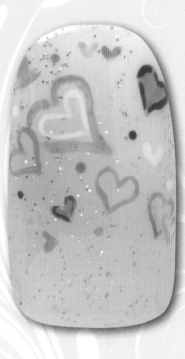

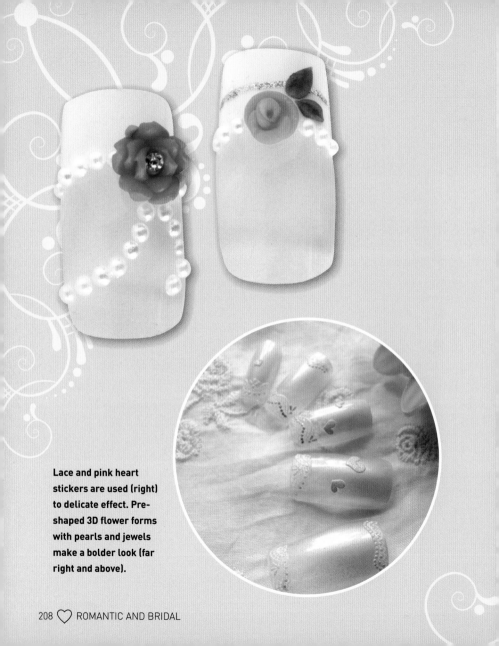

Lace and pink heart
stickers are used (right)
to delicate effect. Pre-
shaped 3D flower forms
with pearls and jewels
make a bolder look (far
right and above).

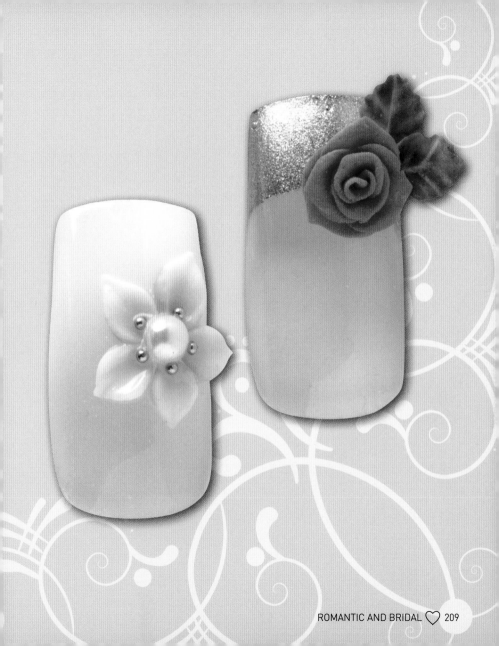

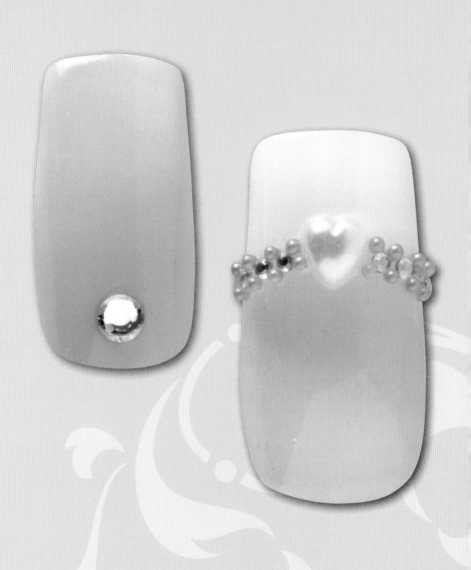

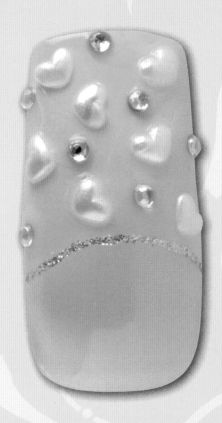

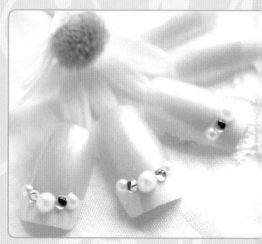

A classic French manicure is given the bridal
treatment with the addition of a row of pearls
and circular rhinestones along the join.

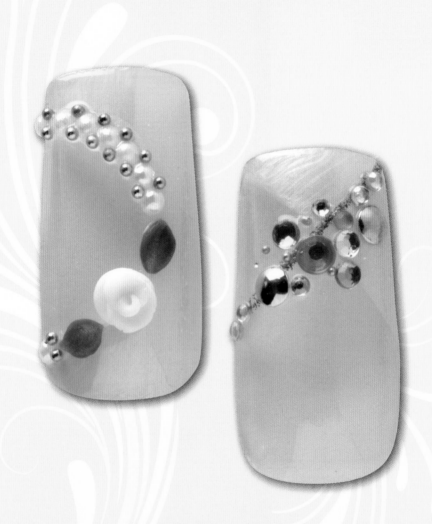

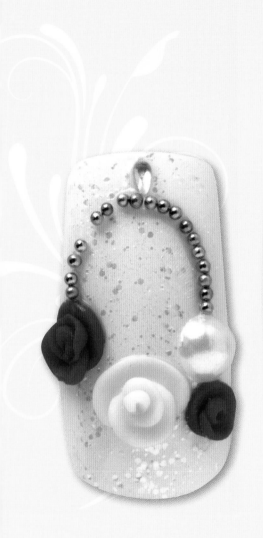
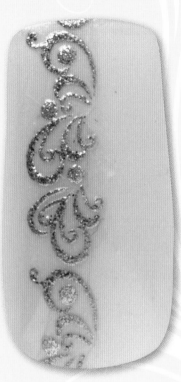

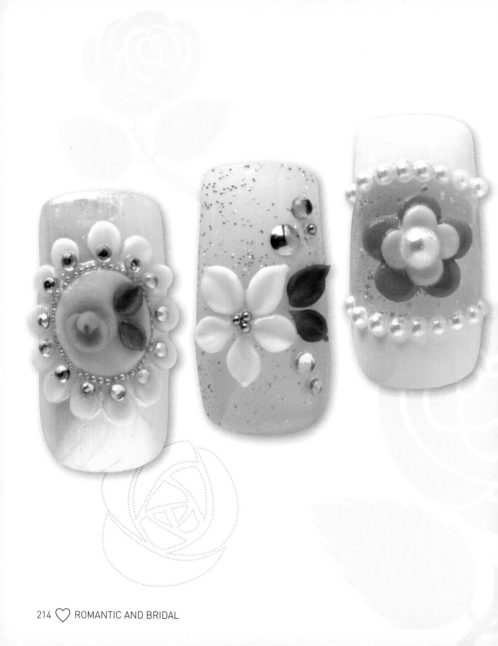

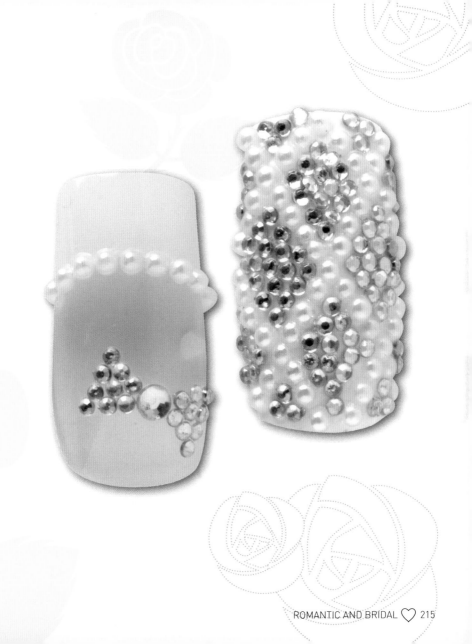

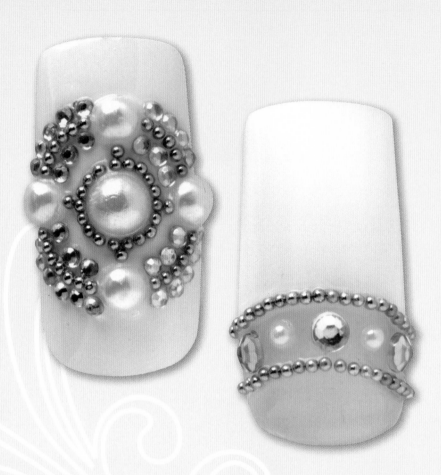

A favourite flower design can be transformed
into a romantic or bridal version by simply
executing the design in white, pink or red –
or perhaps try all three!

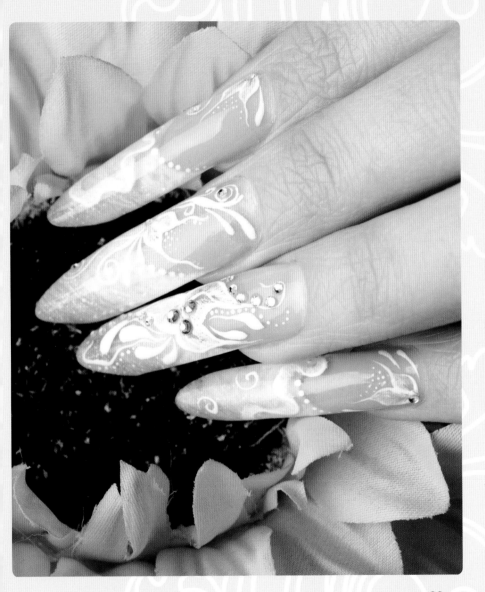

Three-Dimensional Art

Three-dimensional nail art is a relatively recent craze in Europe and the US, but it has been popular for some time in the Far East. It is done by sticking pre-made 3D shapes or stickers onto the nails. They can also be made by manipulating dots and blobs of acrylic gel into different shapes with brushes and/or special-effect tools before they dry. There are also 3D pens available that give the illusion of 3D acrylic gel. The more elaborate versions, often referred to as "stereoscopic" designs, are pre-formed piece by piece, then assembled. These designs are literally "works of art" and can be heavy, which risks damaging the natural nail bed. For this reason they are created on acrylics (fake nails), which are then stuck onto the natural nails.

When creating elaborate, built-up designs, such as flowers, you may need to make each part individually in advance, then assemble them before gluing the finished design onto a coloured nail base. Alternatively, you can pour acrylic mixture into specially-made moulds and turn them out when they are dry. Pre-made shapes are also readily available in a variety of forms from online nail art stores. Flowers are one of the most common three-dimensional creations, although cute animals are also popular. A glitter sealer can look spectacular when applied over a 3D floral design.

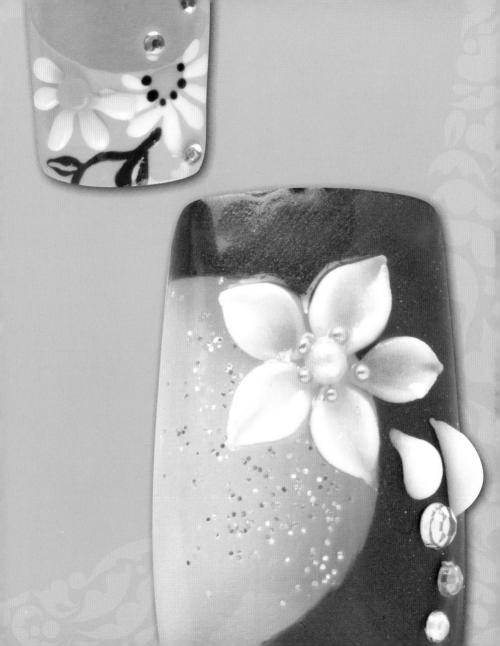

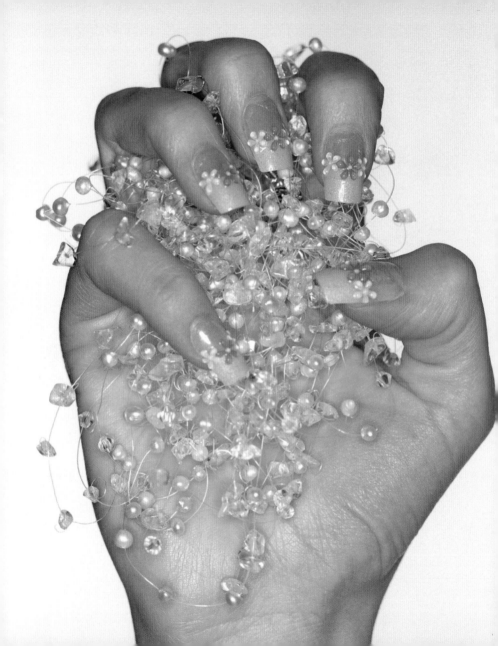

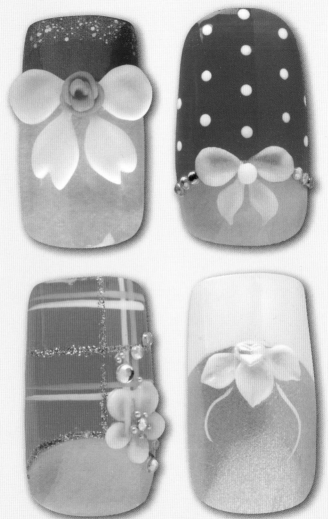

Painted designs can be
enhanced with 3D flower
and bow shapes, combined
with sparkling diamantés.

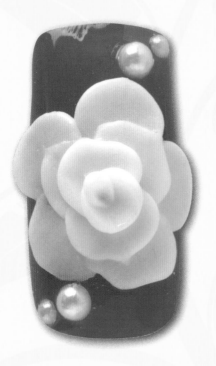
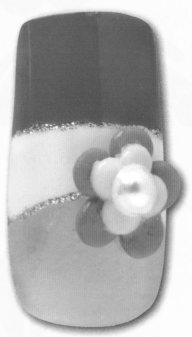

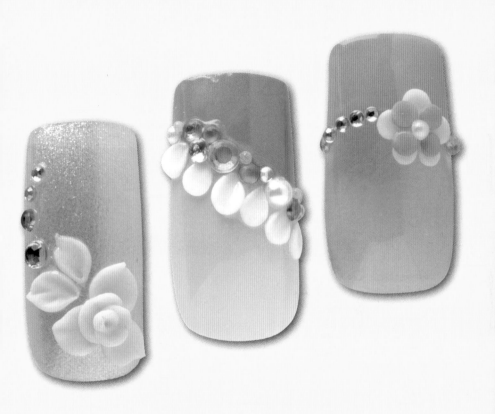

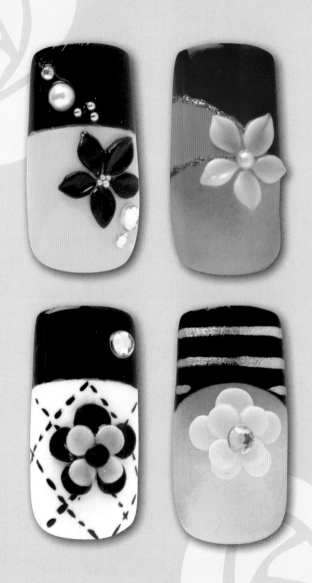

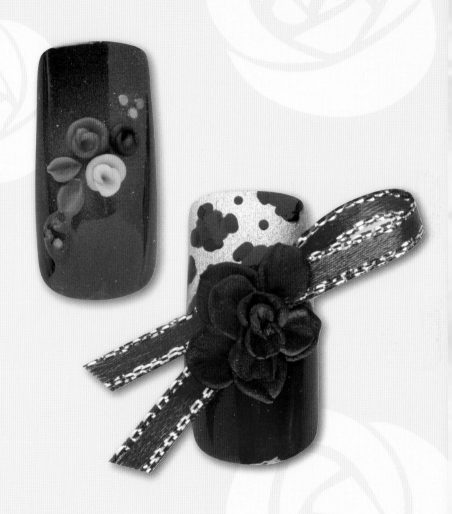

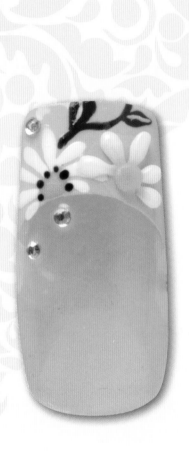
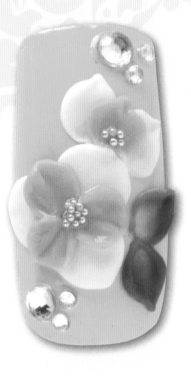

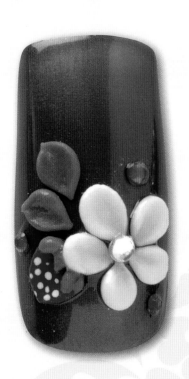
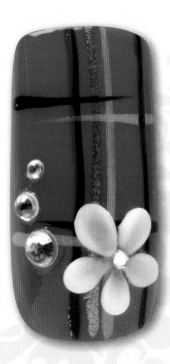

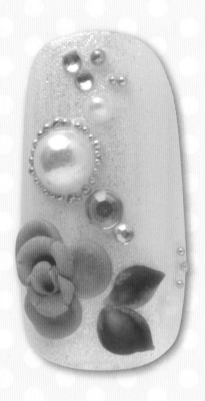
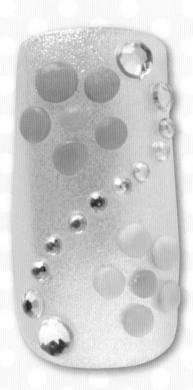

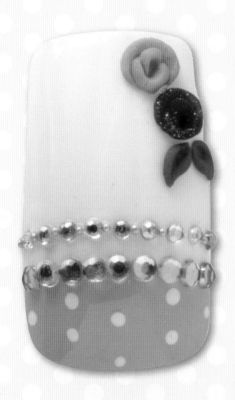
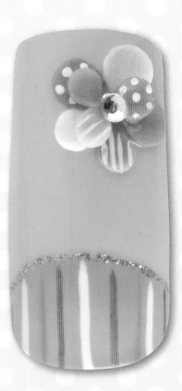

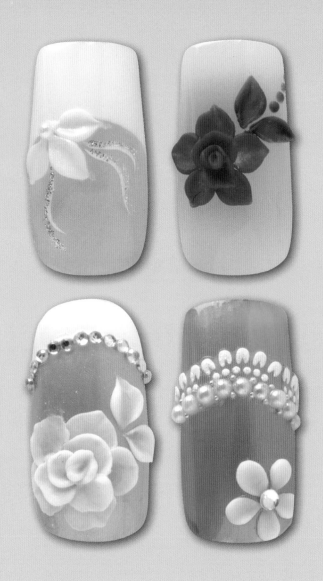

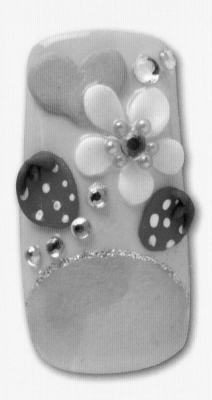
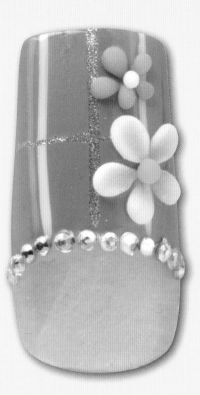

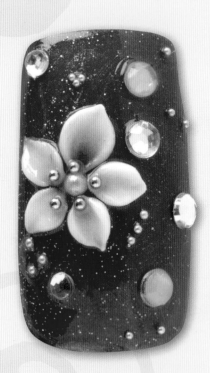
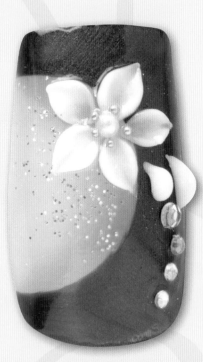

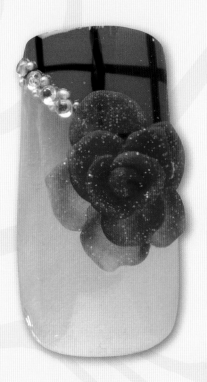
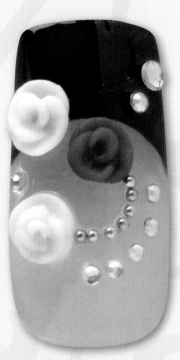

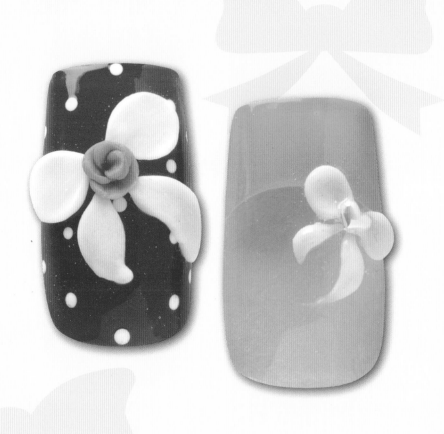

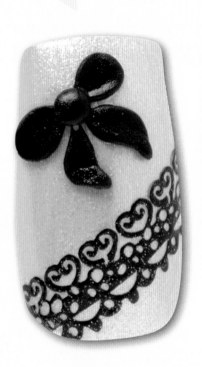
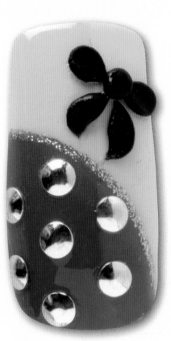

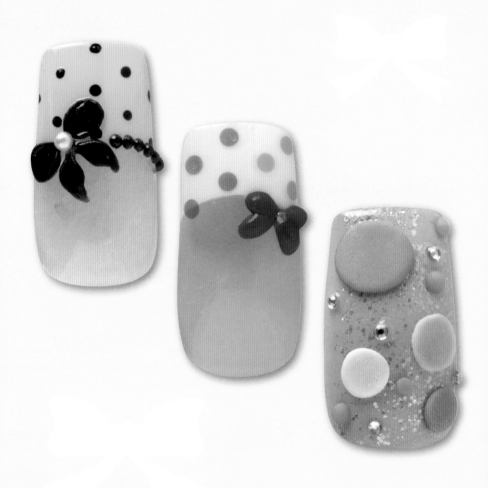

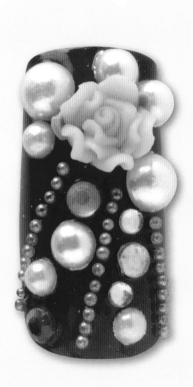
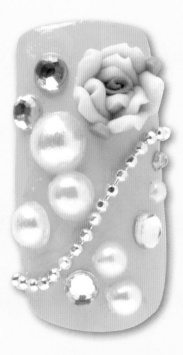

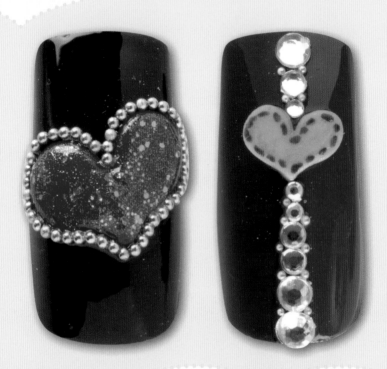

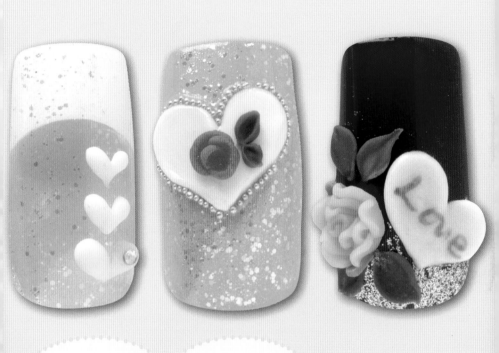

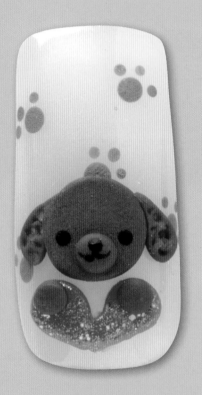
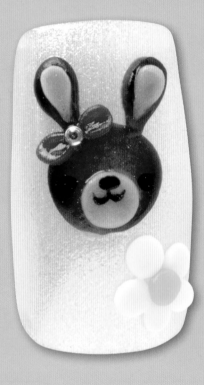
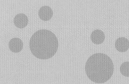

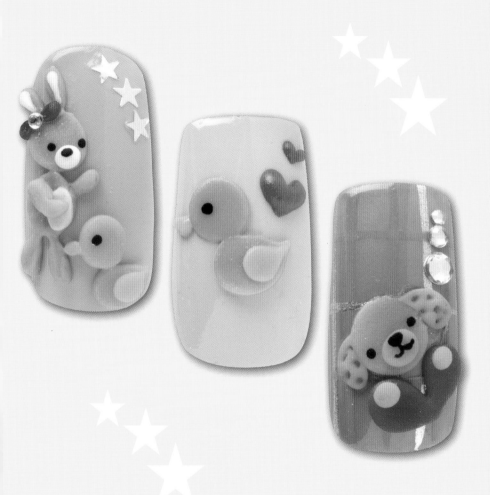

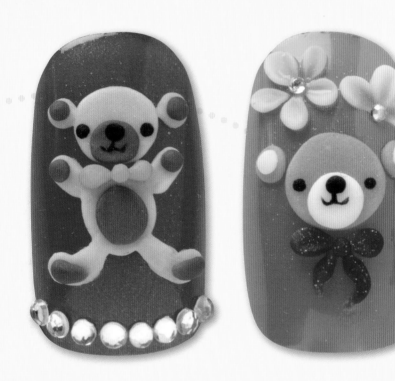

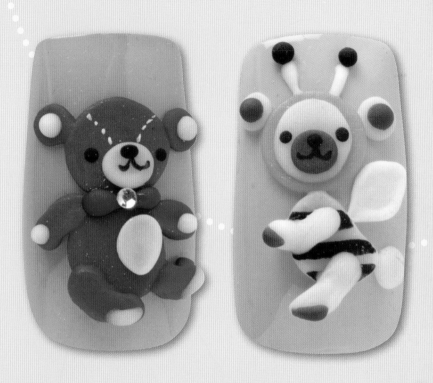

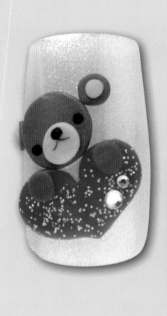
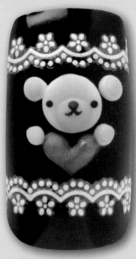
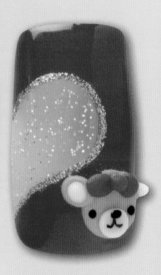

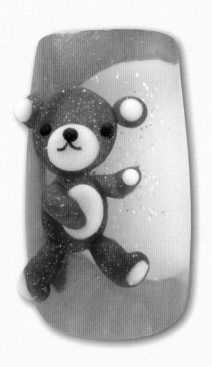
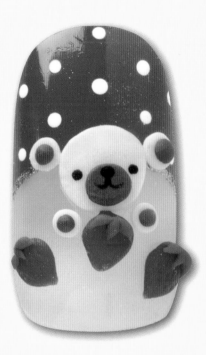
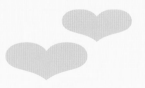

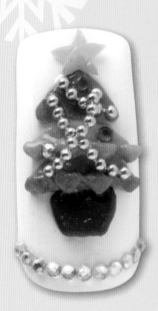
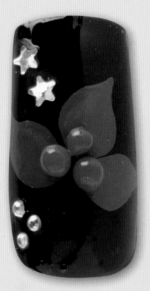
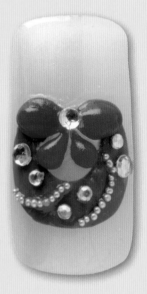

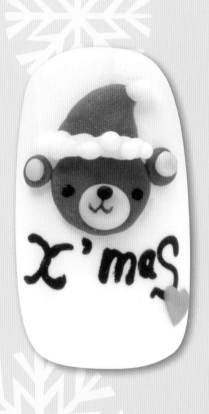
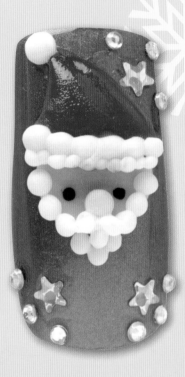

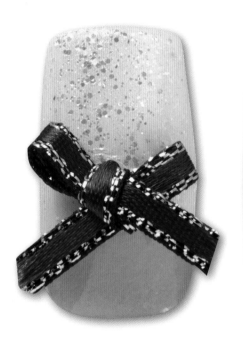
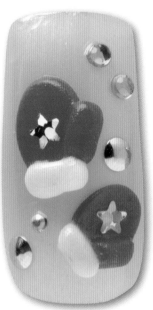

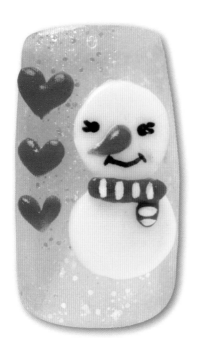
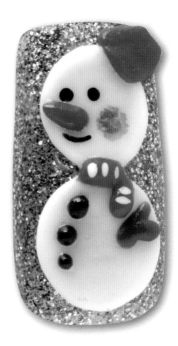

Directory

ARTISTS AND SALONS

UK

Sam Biddle
www.sambiddle.co.uk

Olga Clapcott
Tigerlilly Nails
Beauty in Mind
61d Seamoor Road
Westbourne
Dorset
Tel: 07921 888793
www.olgaclapcott.co.uk

Hazel Dixon
Purely Nailz
10a White Hart Street
Thetford
Norfolk
IP24 1AD
Tel: 01824 766100
www.purelynailz.co.uk

Sarah Gingell
Nail Zone
178 Hope Street
Glasgow G2 2TU
Tel: 0141 332 1999
www.nailzone.co.uk

The Illustrated Nail
Tel: 07816081213
www.theillustratednail.tumblr.com

Julie Nails
289 Kings Road
London SW3 5EW
Tel: 020 735 22251
And also
91–93 Notting Hill Gate
London W11 3JZ
Tel: 020 7243 4188

Gemma Lambert
www.nailangel.co.uk

Jenny Longworth
CLM Hair and Make-up
Top Floor
19 All Saints Road
London W11 1HE
Tel: 020 7313 8330
www.jennylongworth.com

Kirsty Meakin
www.lolnailcourses.com

Megumi Mizuno
M A & D
Vanston Place
London SW6 1AJ
Tel: 07940 707 500
www.maandd.co.uk

Nails Inc
Nail salon chain, visit the website to
find your nearest salon.
www.nailsinc.com

Marianne Newman
www.mariannewmannails.com

Zoe Pocock
Daniel Galvin Jnr
4 West Halkin Street
London SW1X 8JA.
Tel: 02034 163 116
www.danielgalvinjnr.co.uk

Sophy Robson
Hari's Salon
233 Kings Road
London SW3 5EJ
Tel: 020 7349 8722
www.sophyrobson.com

Mineko Sugito
Lapis Lazuli Nails Salon
c/o Cutting Bay Hair Salon
7 Brownlow Road
London N11 2ET
Tel: 07972 722 307

Vikki Taylor-Dodd
Spoilt for Choice
164 Station Rd
Wallsend Ne28 8QT
Tel: 0191 2624357
www.taylordnails.co.uk

Wah Nails
420 Kingsland Road
London E8 4AA
Tel: 020 7812 9889
www.wah-nails.com

Denise Wright
5 Cherry Trees
Hartley
Kent DA3 8DS
Tel: 01474 707077
www.denisewrightatperfect10.co.uk

USA

Athena Elliott
K. Renee Salon
3100 Timmons Ln. #130
Houston TX 77027
www.kreneesalon.com

Kimmie Kyees
Los Angeles, CA
Tel: 6614 378 8252
www.kimmieknails.com

Deborah Lippmann
www.lippmanncollection.com

Erica Marton
425 West 14th St.
3rd Floor
New York, NY 10014
Tel: 212 367 8200
www.faceplace.com

Naja Rickette
Extremedys2012
Hand and Foot Spa
8001 Santa Monica Blvd
West Hollywood CA 90046
Tel: 323-848-8094
www.extremedys2012.com

Fleury Rose
Tomahawk Salon
10 Porter Ave
Brooklyn
Tel: (646) 399-6873.
www.tomahawksalon.com

OTHER
Catherine Wong (Malaysia)
www.ecsalonce.blogspot.com

Cynful Nails (Singapore)
www.cynfulnails.com

SUPPLIERS

SPECIALIST PRODUCTS AND BRANDS:

www.artisticnaildesign.com
Professional gel polish

www.bynubar.com
Healthy, vegan and cruelty-free nail products

www.charm-nails.com
Gels and accessories

www.cuccio.co.uk
Professional nail products

www.dear-laura.com
Nail stickers

www.essie.com
Award-winning nail polish

www.ezflow.com
Professional nail art supplies

www.ibdbeauty.com
Gel polish and accessories

www.jessica-nails.co.uk
Over 200 nail polish colours

www.konadnailart.com
Nail art stamps

www.nailharmony.com
Stockists of Gelish products

www.nailrock.com
Designer nail wraps

www.onenail.net
Galaxy nail products

www.opi.com
Professional quality nail polish

www.orlybeauty.com
Nail products from the inventor
of the French Manicure

www.sallyhansen.co.uk
Nail care products

www.smart-nails.com
Nail stencils

www.sweetsquared.com
Products and nail design courses

GENERAL SUPPLIERS:

www.charismanail.com
General nail art suppliers

www.entitybeauty.com
Professional nail supplies

www.naio.co.uk
Huge Internet store with a wide
rage of nail products

www.naildelights.com
General nail product suppliers,
worldwide shipping

www.nailtechsupply.com
US-based nail product suppliers

www.nailtopia.co.uk
Nail art products including glitter, gems and stickers

www.premiumnails.com
Professional nail products

www.professionalnailsupplies.co.uk
Large stock of nail supplies including imported products

www.vivalanails.co.uk
Vast range of nail art supplies, including nail art canes, water decals and rhinestones

INTERNET TUTORIALS AND VIDEOS

Many of the main brands and suppliers have tutorials on their websites. You Tube is also a good source for step-by-step tutorials:

You Tube: Cute Polish
You Tube: Viva la Nails
You Tube: Cuteglitternails
You Tube: EliszaNails

COURSES

Many nail brands also run courses in how to use their products, see their websites for details.

Confederation of International Beauty Therapy and Cosmetology (CIBTAC)
www.cibtac.com
Internationally recognized beauty qualifications

MAGAZINES

Scratch Magazine
www.scratchmagazine.co.uk
UK-based nail magazine

Nails Magazine
www.nailsmag.com
US-based nail magazine

Nailpro
www.nailpro.com
US-based nail magazine

Acknowledgements

The publishers would to like to thank the following sources for their kind permission to reproduce the pictures in this book.

Key: t=Top, b=Bottom, c=Centre, l=Left and r=Right

Alamy: /Ruzanna Arutyunyan: 168, / Serg Zastavkin: 141

Camera Press: 152, 162, 165, 220

Corbis: /Herry Choi /TongRo Image Stock: 15r, 146, /Imagemore Co. Ltd.: 14, /Sonja Pacho: 64, 72, / Hiroshi Watanabe /amanaimages: 26l, 48, 59t, 68, 115l, 122r, 123c, 123r, 126, 129b, /Adrianna Williams: 124–125, /Becky Yee: 79

Getty Images: /Henry Beeker, Age Fotostock, Photolibrary UK: 102, / Naho Yoshizawa, Aflo Foto Agency, Photolibrary UK: 197

istockphoto.com: /A1ex76: 21, 39r, /Dean Bertoncelj: 2–3, 116, 117, / coloroftime: 34, 217, /Gisele: 101, /Jodi Jacobson: 7, /jreika: 208b, 211r, /Zoia Kostina: 154, /Ivan Mateev: 156b, /Andrey Popov: 37

SuperStock: /© Fotosearch: 15l

Thinkstock: /Hemera: 4–5, 26r, 29, 30, 31, 46, 46–47, 67b, 74, 86, 90, 91, 92, 93, 95, 96, 98, 100, 103, 105, 106, 108, 111, 167r, 169t, 170b, 171l, /istockphoto: 16t, 16b, 43, 49, 51, 52, 62, 84, 87, 88, 89, 108–109, 110, 112–113, 138, 148, 155, 158, 159, 166–167, 181

All other images © Carlton Books.

Every effort has been made to acknowledge correctly and contact the source and/or copyright holder of each picture and Carlton Books Limited apologizes for any unintentional errors or omissions, which will be, corrected in future editions of this book.